The *back to eden* Cookbook ®

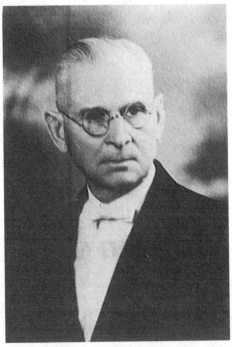

Jethro Kloss, pioneer advocate of returning to nature for health and healing. Master nutritionist, he had an instinctive genius for tasteful, healthful cookery.

The
back to eden
Cookbook

The JETHRO KLOSS Family
Promise Kloss Moffett and Doris Kloss Gardiner

ॐ

Original recipes and nutritional information from one of
the great pioneers in the imaginative use of natural foods.

Illustrated by Daniel Guild

BACK TO EDEN BOOKS
®

Published and Distributed by

BACK TO EDEN BOOKS
P.O. Box 1439
Loma Linda, California 92354

Library of Congress Catalog Card Number 81-82412

International Standard Book Number 0-940676-03-6

Printed in the United States of America.

Contents

Jethro Kloss . . . Pioneer Nutritionist ... 7

Return To Eden . . . Return To Happiness ... 11

Soy Milk, Cheese, Butter, and Cream ... 35

Nut Milk, Cheese, Butter, and Cream ... 41

Main Dishes ... 45

Using Sprouted Seeds ... 61

Bread . . . a Health Food ... 65

Life-Giving Breads ... 74

Natural Breakfast Foods ... 87

Soups . . . Total Nutrition ... 94

Salads and Dressings ... 105

Vegetables ... 115

Sauces, Seasonings, and Spreads ... 129

Desserts for Health ... 136

Coffees, Teas, and Broths ... 149

Index ... 156

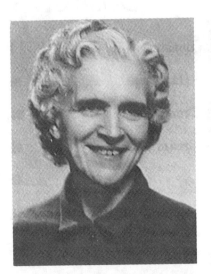

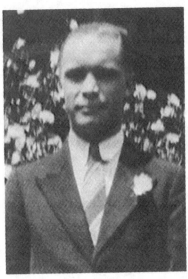

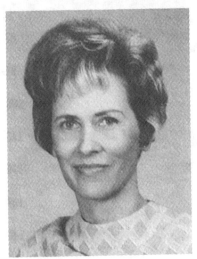

THE KLOSS FAMILY

Dedicated to continuing the life work and philosophy of Jethro Kloss... his daughter, Promise Kloss Moffett (above left); his granddaughter, Doris Kloss Gardiner (lower left); and his son, Eden Kloss.

Jethro Kloss
... Pioneer Nutritionist

—an introduction by his daughter

By PROMISE KLOSS MOFFETT

An editor of **Prevention** magazine has described my father as a crusader for better health, one of the early pioneers, one of the most famous of the herbal healers.

All this he surely was — and a man warm-hearted and affectionate, wholly dedicated to helping others.

His classic work, **Back To Eden** (Back To Eden Books), is a summary of his half a century of experience in using natural remedies and natural foods for healing as well as for maintaining health.

Jethro Kloss was a master cook and baker, as can be testified to by members of the Kloss family who worked with him through his years of study, experimentation, and teaching.

From his earliest childhood on a pioneer farm in Wisconsin, my father and his parents made nature their study and with great ingenuity developed effective and attractive ways of using the natural products of the soil. This inquiring and inventive attitude he maintained throughout his life.

He was firm in a reverent belief in God and the Edenic plan that man eat of fruits, grains, nuts, and vegetable products rather than refined or synthetic materials, or animals or animal products.

He was one of the earliest developers of vegetarian meat substitutes prepared with an outstanding sense of eye and taste appeal.

A true "evangelist" for the natural life, for natural foods, Jethro Kloss had a sense of showmanship and produced such programs as his remarkable "Demonstration Dinners" in Washington, D.C., in the 1930's. At these beautifully arranged events, attended by many Washington notables, my father showed people how attractive and tasteful a truly healthful meal could be.

As early as the 1910's and 1920's, Jethro Kloss operated a series of health food factories from which a great variety of natural foods were made available at reasonable prices to people throughout the country and throughout the world.

His inventive mind was always trying to find a new and better way. He originated many new foods but was constantly experimenting, improving. He never seemed to rest satisfied, but would continue to try for a finer texture, a more delicate flavor, or perhaps a better method of preserving nutritional values in cooking or preserving food.

My father felt a kinship with nature and reveled in its beauty and its bounty. I think I never knew a person who more keenly enjoyed the good things of life. When he was nearing the end of his dedicated and active life of service he visited my husband and me in southern British Columbia. Near our house a little stream dashed white down the steep rocks from mountain springs above. I can see him yet catching the sparkling water in his tin cup, then drinking deeply of its refreshing coolness. He enjoyed working in our garden and how he delighted in the varied flavors of its fruits and vegetables!

We urged him to stay with us but he could not settle down. He felt that he must hasten back to accomplish more for "suffering humanity." That expression was a favorite of his. His heart was greatly touched when someone told him of pain or illness and he was always anxious to alleviate it.

He went peacefully to sleep at last in his 84th year and now rests in a little cemetery in Tennessee awaiting what he fervently believed would be a certain resurrection at the return of Jesus Christ.

His host of friends and all the beneficiaries of his life of dedicated service will perpetuate his memory. And in the continuing family publication of his book, **Back To Eden,** and now in **The Back To Eden Cookbook,** we his children and heirs are resolved to make his knowledge and the devout spirit of his work available to people throughout the world in their search for the better life.

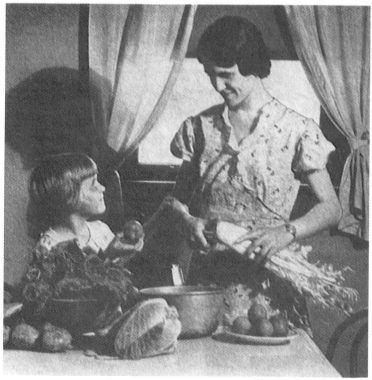

Promise Kloss Moffett and her niece, Doris Kloss Gardiner who was Jethro's only grandchild. (Published in Life and Health *in August, 1934.)*

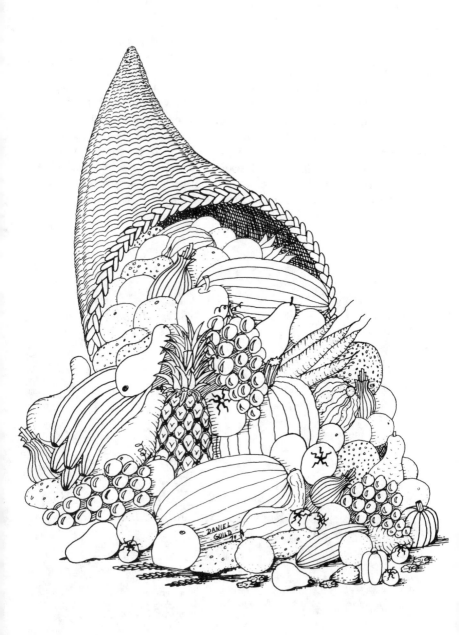

Return To Eden
...Return To Happiness

It is recorded in the Bible that our first parents lived an unblemished life in a Garden of Eden.

In this paradise, the record says, the Creator of this universe made man in the very beginning out of the ground itself.

And it is true that the different properties found in the earth are also found in man and that fruits, grains, nuts, and vegetables contain the same elements which are in the earth, and in man.

When these fruits, grains, nuts, and vegetables are eaten in their natural state and not perverted and robbed of their life-giving properties by careless preparation, health, beauty and happiness will be the sure reward.

God in his infinite wisdom neglected nothing, and if we would eat our food without trying to improve, change, and refine it, thereby destroying its life-giving elements, it would meet all requirements of a healthful existence.

Returning is Renewing

Today, I believe that our health depends on how nearly we return to a state of harmony with nature's laws; on how nearly we return in principle and practice to the life of Eden. An all-wise God put within nature all the elements necessary for the building of our bodies. It is wrong habits of eating and the use of refined and adulterated foods that are largely responsible for the intemperance, crime, and sickness that curse this world.

The results of man's trying to improve on nature is a deterioration of the human race — especially in countries where people are accustomed to so-called luxuries. Although food may be ample in quantity, modern methods of refining remove the most important elements and in many cases the foods are adulterated with preservatives, flavorings, and colorings to conceal inferior nutritional quality.

A True Diet

A true diet is not based on calories but on the organic elements that give and sustain life. Our most common and serious deseases are caused by wrong eating and drinking. This has been proven by numerous scientific experiments in recent years. Food is a substance that, when absorbed by the bloodstream, will nourish, repair, and furnish life-force and heat to the body. But if in its preparation and refining the life-giving elements are taken away, it cannot furnish life force but will distort the functional activity of the body and result in many disorders.

Actually, many diseases are nature's effort to free our system of poisons and congestions resulting from wrong eating and drinking. When we assist nature in expelling impurities and re-establishing right conditions in the system we can overcome disease.

The whole world needs more vitamins, better cooks, more care exercised in the preparation of food and less spacious hospitals.

Since Eve first surrendered to appetite, man has been growing more and more self-indulgent until health is being sacrificed on the altar of appetite. How strange — when God Himself gave our first parents ideal foods designed specifically for the human race!

No Meat in Man's Original Diet

The Bible tells us that man's original diet did not include meats or animal products.

Today, meat eating is becoming more and more dangerous because of the steady increase in disease among animals. Some time ago I had a nice herd of registered Jerseys. One morning we noticed in the paper that in the adjoining county they had to kill thousands of cattle on account of disease. I decided to sell my stock and keep only three of the best milk cows.

About six or eight months later, a neighbor said to me one morning, "Did you hear that Anderson had 16 cows die yesterday and couldn't do anything for them?" Then I decided to sell two of my three cows and just keep "old Lizzie," a registered Jersey. Her milk tested 6½ percent butter fat. She had never had anything but the very best of feed and the very best of care possible.

Still, a few weeks later she became sick and refused all food. I told my wife not to use the milk for a day or two, hoping there would be a change for the better but there was none. Old Lizzie walked as if she were afraid to step on her feet and made queer movements with her lower jaw. All at once she fell over and was dead. We decided then that we would never use any more milk.

Some time after this we noticed that there were four or five states in which the chickens as well as the cows were so diseased that for a long time they were not permitted to ship any eggs or butter or livestock. While we had not used any milk for a long time prior to this, we then stopped using all milk, meat, or eggs and have not used them since. We have found an abundance of good things to take their place.

A few years prior to this I was up in the northern states near the clearwater lakes and found millions of fish dead on the water. On being examined they were found to have a live worm along the spine which killed them.

Not long ago, while in San Diego, California, I was told by reliable persons that not far from San Diego the dead fish were so thick on the water that ships had a hard time to move through them.

No Need for Animal Products

For many years I have spent much money and time to produce articles of food which most perfectly take the place of meat, milk, eggs, and butter. These articles are very palatable, are easily digested, furnish perfect nourishment, and are very inexpensive — costing only a fraction of the amount paid for animal products. You will find all of them in this book.

Facts About Food

If all the refined breakfast foods and baked products on the market should be discarded and people would make their own bread from whole grain flour, not only would their expenses be much less but they would also prevent a great deal of suffering and doctor bills.

White flour bread cannot impart to the system the nourishment that will be found in whole grain bread. The use of fine flour aggravates difficulties for those who have ineffective livers.

Most of the "whole wheat" breads purchased in the stores are unhealthful because they contain various percentages of white flour and are seldom baked enough. Bread is more healthful when it is at least one day old. It should be baked clear through so that not any part of it is soft or gummy.

Benefits of a Raw Diet

I believe in eating everything in its raw and natural state as far as possible — at least of the foods that can be easily digested. I once read an article by a man who thought we should never cook anything but eat it raw as people did in the beginning of time. But this fact is generally overlooked: foods are not as they were in the beginning.

In the beginning, the Bible says, fruits, grains, and nuts grew all the year around and there was no need to can, cook, and bake as there is today. The wheat, rye, barley, oats, beans, and nuts were never hard and dry as they are now.

Fresh fruits and grains were eaten in their milky or grape-sugar state, in which they needed scarcely any digestion — like our green corn.

That is something I like to eat — green corn, plump with its own fresh milk. It is then in the grape-sugar state and easily digested. It requires very little cooking. After it matures and gets dry it has entered a starchy state and no man has a digestive fluid with which to digest raw starch. Therefore we need to grind and bake it. If properly baked, the starch again becomes grape-sugar.

Too Much Protein

Much impurity is produced in the system by too much protein. Now we know how to prepare our food and what foods to eat in order to balance the amount of protein with other foods, so as to avoid overtaxing the system with too much protein.

Corn, wheat, peas, and beans in their milky state — before they are full-grown — contain only 3 to 4 percent protein but are high in minerals and other life-giving properties. When they mature, the wheat has from 8 to 14 percent protein, the dried corn a little less, while the beans have from 20 to 30 percent or more.

All beans, lentils, and corn may be picked and canned in the milky state. Being thus very low in protein, everyone can eat freely of them.

Sprouting for High Food Value

Peas, beans, lentils, and grains can be sprouted (see section on sprouting), turning the protein into pure peptones, amino acids, to a great extent and the starches and sugars into dextrose and grape sugar. They are then very easy to digest. Also, the sprouts have a very good flavor and are higher in many life-giving properties than the original seed.

Leafy vegetables such as spinach, lettuce, celery, and cabbage are good taken in their raw, natural state.

Fresh, cleanly prepared raw vegetable juices are excellent for supplying the body with natural minerals, salts, and vitamins. It is necessary that the vegetables be properly macerated so that the life elements are released into the liquid.

Time Required for Digestion

Rice, boiled .... 1 hr	Bread, corn, baked ... 3¼ hrs
Barley, boiled .... 2 hrs	Apples, hard and sour,
Milk, boiled .... 2 hrs	raw .... 3 hrs
Milk (raw) .... 2½ hrs	Apples, sweet and
Egg (soft boiled) .... 3 hrs	mellow, raw ...... 2 hrs
Egg (hard boiled) .... 3½ hrs	Parsnips, boiled ..... 2½ hrs
Egg (fried) .... 3½ hrs	Carrots, boiled ...... 3¼ hrs
Egg (raw) .... 2 hrs	Beets, boiled .... 3¾ hrs
Butter .... 3½ hrs	Turnips, boiled ...... 3½ hrs
Green corn and beans,	Potatoes, Irish,
boiled .... 3¾ hrs	baked .... 2½ hrs
Vegetable hash,	Potatoes, Irish,
warmed .... 2½ hrs	boiled .... 3½ hrs
Bread, whole wheat,	Cabbage, raw .... 2½ hrs
baked .... 3½ hrs	Cabbage, boiled .... 4½ hrs

Cooking for Life

More care must be exercised in cooking food so as not to destroy its vitamins, minerals, and other life-giving properties.

Much good food is ruined in preparation and more which is not ruined in preparation becomes detrimental because it is served in too many varieties and often in too large quantities. Thus, acids, gases, and fermentation are set up, spoiling the food after it is eaten and keeping it from making good blood.

Foods improperly prepared lose much of their food value. I repeat, it is very essential that foods be eaten in the natural state as much as possible. Too much cooking is injurious. Certain elements are destroyed by even a small amount of heat and for that reason such foods as can be eaten raw should be served often. Green, leafy vegetables such as cabbage, spinach, romaine, dandelion, carrots, lettuce, endive, celery and many others contain those substances that the human body must have to function properly. A lack of such elements in the diet is a kind of starvation and will end disastrously.

Such vegetables as carrots, tender beets, parsnips, cucumbers, potatoes, or young turnips should not be peeled. The highest mineral content of such foods lies just under the skins and, therefore, is lost if they are peeled.

Neither should any of the water from vegetables be thrown away. It contains valuable mineral salts and should be used. In cooking leafy vegetables, just enough water should be added to keep them from burning and they should not be cooked longer than is absolutely necessary.

For example, spinach or beet tops should never be cooked over eight or ten minutes. If beets are cooked with tops (it takes much longer to cook the beets than the tops), the beets should be diced fine and cooked with only enough water to keep them from burning. Use the stems but cut in quarter-inch lengths, adding them after the beets are about half-done (about 30 minutes). Cut the leaves fine and when the beets are about done, add the leaves for it takes only a few minutes (about 10) to cook them. The salt should be added after the stems have come to a boil and a little Soy Butter (see recipe) diluted with water to the consistency of cream added just

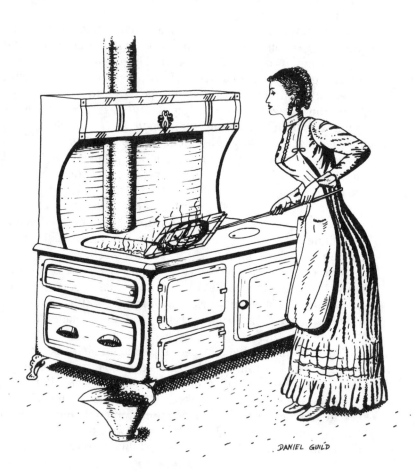

DANIEL GUILD

as the heat is turned off — or it can be added when the dish is served.

Never put soda in your vegetables to tender them or brighten the color. Neither should soda be used in cooking dried peas, beans, corn, etc., even if it does shorten the cooking time. Moreover, the common use of soda biscuits and corn bread made with baking powder and soda can be the cause of various deficiency diseases because it destroys much of the vitamin content of foods. Remember that disease cannot get a foothold when the body is in a healthy condition.

Cooking for Easier Digestion

Food must be prepared properly to be well-digested and thoroughly assimilated. Our physical well-being depends on this. Ninety percent of all human ills originate in the stomach and are caused from overeating, wrong combinations of food, and unnatural foods.

Food properly cooked is always easily digested.

All food should be prepared in one of the following ways: boiled, steamed, broiled, baked, stewed, braised, roasted, or simmered. Do not use fried foods, except when you wish to warm up something in a frying pan — and then it does not need to be fried hard. Fried foods are indigestible — poisonous to the system.

The best way to cook vegetables is to bake them. Boiling is good if just enough water is used for cooking and none thrown away. Waterless cooking, casserole baking, and low-pressure steam cooking are also good.

When cooking vegetables in water, start with boiling water, no more than enough to cook the vegetables. If any water remains, save it and add it to your soups or broths. The vegetables must boil continuously after starting; otherwise they will become water-soaked. It is not necessary for them to boil hard; only moderately.

Add salt in moderation just before the vegetables are entirely done. Salt added at the beginning tends to toughen foods. Do not overcook vegetables; only until tender—

overcooking destroys the life-giving properties. Do not add fats to vegetables when cooking; add seasonings just before the vegetables are done and serve at once.

Never peel or remove the eyes from Irish potatoes before cooking; the life of the potato is in the eyes and peeling. Do not peel any vegetable that can be used without peeling. Carrots, parsnips, salsify, rutabagas, and others may be scraped thinly so as not to lose the minerals, which are just under their skins.

Green vegetables are very desirable during the winter months. If you think them expensive, remember that they are far cheaper than the cost of sickness; and, when they are properly prepared, are real medicine.

Canned vegetables are not as good as fresh vegetables properly prepared; but if you get a good brand, they are better than fresh vegetables poorly prepared.

Vegetables can be seasoned with Soy Mayonnaise, leaving out the lemon (see recipe). Dilute it with cold water to the consistency of cream or you can use as is. Rich soy milk or one of the nut milks are good when added to hot vegetables (see recipes). Heat only a few minutes after milk has been added and serve at once. Good soy milk can now be purchased, so you can always have it on hand.

Eat all the non-starchy vegetables raw if they agree with you; such as carrots, cabbage, cucumbers, radishes, and parsley.

Alkaline food should comprise 75 to 95 percent of the everyday diet. If you have any ailments your diet should be at least 90 percent alkaline, base-forming foods. Acid foods bring on diseases while alkaline foods help to overcome and even to prevent disease.

Here are some examples of acid foods:

Starch foods	White rice
Creamed potatoes	Cornstarch pudding
Macaroni	White crackers
Spaghetti	Chicken dumplings
White bread	Demineralized cereals
Biscuits	

Timetable for Cooking

Apples, sour	medium-hot oven	30 min.
Apples, sweet	medium-hot oven	45 min.
Asparagus	boiled	20 min.
Beets	boiled	until tender
Carrots	boiled	until tender
Cauliflower	boiled	until tender
Whole cereals	direct boiling	1 hr.
	double boiler	2-4 hrs.
Cookies	moderate oven	8 to 15 min.
Corn, green	boiled	2 to 3 min.
Dried beans	boiled until tender, then bake	
Eggplant	baked — hot oven	30 min.
Muffins	quick oven	25 min.
Oats	direct boiling	45 min.
	double boiler	1 hr.
Onions	boiled	until tender
Parsnips	boiled	45-60 min.
Peas	boiled	until tender
Potatoes	baked — hot oven	45-60 min.
Potatoes	boiled	35-45 min.
Rice	boiled	20-30 min.
Whole grain rolls and biscuits	quick oven	20-25 min.
Salsify	boiled	2 hrs.
Squash	boiled	until well done
String beans	boiled	until tender
Sweet potatoes	baked, hot oven	45 min.
Tomatoes	boiled	10-15 min.
Turnips	boiled	until tender

The Best Protein Sources

Proteins are tissue-builders and absolutely indispensable. There is a high-quality protein content in soybeans, which makes them a successful substitute for meat, milk, and eggs. They contain double the amount of protein found in beefsteak. They are the only natural food in the vegetable kingdom that contains higher protein nutritive values than meat, milk, and eggs.

Extensive experiments have shown that one can eat,

without ill effects, at least three times more soybean protein than meat.

The soybean, in fact, has life-giving properties which meat and other protein foods do not have.

Increasing knowledge of the value of the soybean is one of the greatest nutritional developments in history.

Anyone with a piece of ground may grow his own soybeans. They will not only greatly improve the soil and make virgin soil out of worn-out soil but at the same time they will supply 'a family with the most delicious and nourishing food. Soybeans should be planted at intervals throughout the spring in order to have shelled soybeans all summer. The green soybeans can be shelled just like any other bean or pea. Some varieties that do not shell easily can be helped by first boiling for just a few minutes.

Soy milk can be made from soybeans at home for pennies a quart. The Yellow Mammoth, Dixie, Illinois, and Tokyo soybeans are among the best varieties for soy milk but there are other varieties better for green shelled beans.

For stomach ulcers, duodenal ulcers, cancer and diabetes; as well as for liver, kidney, and bladder troubles, soy milk is not only a good food but also a real medicine. It is easily digested, does not curd, is highly alkaline, and is rich in minerals.

The soybean is one of the greatest and most complete of foods. In the Orient, it has been used for thousands of years. In this country it has been used for some time for stockfeed and to improve the milk, but only recently has much effort been made to use it for human consumption. At the present time, there are many persons and organizations developing its potential — and with considerable success.

The objection to the soybean is that, for some persons, it does not have a flavor as pleasant as some of the other beans. However, the flavor can be improved by preparing the beans in a different way for human consumption. I have experimented with soybeans for 15 years and have produced a fine, acceptable soy milk as well as many other soybean products.

In fact, I use soybeans in some 50 dishes! I make a soybean bread, buns, pie, pones, roast, cottage cheese, soy cheese (very similar to cream cheese or American yellow cheese). I also make soybean coffee and ice cream. I use no refined sugar in any of these products.

My soy milk is simply delicious—very palatable, and children like it as well as adults.

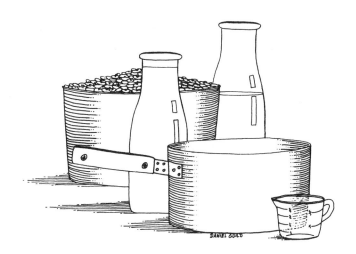

Delicious Soy Milk

Soy milk properly made is a wonderful food for the sick. It does not form hard curds in the stomach and putrify as does cows or goats milk and can be used in the same ways they are used.

Beans and peas cook more quickly when they are boiled in soy milk than when boiled in water. Soy milk will sour and clabber like cows milk and, after souring, can be beaten up into most delicious buttermilk.

The beauty of it is that it is highly alkaline and is well-adapted to the human system — for both adults and children.

Many pay a big price for goats milk while soy milk is infinitely better for human consumption. It does not have the contamination of the animal in it nor the liability to disease and putrefaction.

Here is an analysis of human, cows, goats, soy and nut milk:

Milk	Water	Ash	Protein	Fat	Carbohydrates
	%	%	%	%	%
Human	89.95	0.25	1.30	2.50	6.00
Cows	87.30	0.80	3.20	3.50	5.20
Goats	87.00	0.50	4.00	4.50	4.00
Soy	87.03	2.52	2.40	3.15	6.90
Nut	87.00	2.03	5.60	5.50	7.23

To the soy milk used for the above analysis, I added a little emulsified soybean oil and a little malt.

See the recipe sections of this book for directions that will help you to use soy milk and its products in all the ways one would use cows milk.

Vegetable Juices

Carrot juice — Is rich in vitamins, is antiseptic, an alkalinizer, normalizes the blood. Good for anemia, skin troubles, eyes, malnutrition, chronic infection, acidosis, helps to gain weight and aids in overcoming digestive disorders.

Celery juice — Is a solvent rich in vitamins, alkaline. Good for arthritis and other rheumatic troubles, nervous disorders, heart diseases, indigestion, colds, hardening of the arteries, and skin diseases.

Cabbage juice — Antiseptic, cleanser, great help in removing toxins from the system. Good for poor elimination, toxemia, and intestinal putrefaction.

Cucumber juice — Is good for the nerves, a cleanser and diuretic. Good for cleansing the body of toxins; good for nerves, kidneys, and bladder.

Spinach juice — Very rich in vitamins, a blood builder, and alkaline. Good for constipation, chronic infections, anemia, glandular trouble; rich in iron.

Parsley juice — Laxative, blood builder, detoxicant. Good for gallstones, gas, elimination, anemia; a blood builder.

Lettuce juice — Rich in vitamins, alkaline, aids digestion, diuretic. Good for kidney disorders, goiter, lung trouble, ulcers anywhere in the body, and nerves.

Beet juice — Alkaline, good for nerves. Good for anemia, allaying fevers, a blood builder. Use the small, young beets — leaves and all.

Tomato juice — Very rich in vitamins, alkaline. Good for acidosis, infections, liver, kidneys, anemia. Tomato juice belongs with the fruit juices — the acid juices.

Watercress juice — Vitamins, alkaline, a blood builder. Good for anemia, rheumatism, and infections.

Vegetable juices may be mixed. In fact, some of them have to be mixed as they are too strong taken alone.

Carrot, celery, and parsley juices mixed are very good. Mix equal parts of carrot and celery juice and one tablespoon parsley juice to the glass.

Carrot and celery juice are very good for the nerves and general health. Celery juice is excellent for arthritis.

Raw potassium broth, made from celery, spinach, carrot, and parsley juice, supplies nearly all the organic minerals and salts necessary.

Carrot juice alone is wonderful in ulcerous and cancerous conditions. It is also good for the eyes and the respiratory organs generally and increases vigor and vitality.

Carrot and beet juice is a good combination. Beets are very rich in sodium and help to cleanse the system of inorganic calcium. Also good for hardening of the arteries or thickening of the blood which cause high blood pressure. Add cucumber juice to carrot and beet juice and you have a wonderfully fine cleanser as well as health material for the gall bladder, liver, kidneys, and the prostate and other sex glands. This combination of juice is said to dissolve gallstones and kidney stones in a short time.

Carrot and cabbage juices cleanse the mucous membrane of the stomach and are good for pyorrhea.

A sauce made of carrot radish and horseradish makes a cleanser of body mucous. This will cleanse the sinus and the entire body of mucous.

Lettuce juice is very rich in iron (one of the most important elements in the body). When combined with carrot juice it is even better. A combination of carrot, spinach, and lettuce juice is valuable for the hair and nerves. It stimulates the growth of hair.

Spinach juice is a very important juice, especially for the digestive tract. It furnishes the finest organic element to cleanse the rebuilding organs of digestion and overcomes constipation in a natural way.

How To Use Some Fruit Juices

Lemon juice — Very rich source of vitamin C; antiseptic, alkaline, and tonic. Good for nerves, eyes, kidneys. Helps dropsy, high blood pressure, catarrhs, rheumatism, arthritis. Cleanses outside and inside.

Grapefruit juice — Alkaline, many vitamins, laxative. Excellent for constipation, blood diseases, nerves, sleeplessness (taken hot upon retiring), acidosis, and colds.

Grapefruit bitters — Made by grinding or chopping fine the whole grapefruit — peeling, pulp, fruit, and seeds; cover with water and allow to stand overnight. Pour off the liquid and drink — hot or cold. Especially good for throat congestion, colds, sluggish digestion, and infections.

Orange juice — Very rich in vitamins; is alkaline. Excellent tonic; good for digestive weakness, acidosis, sluggish digestion, catarrh, and liver.

I do not recommend that anyone try to live on juices but they are good to drink between meals. Use only one fruit juice at a time.

The Value of a Fruit Diet

Nearly all fruits contain acids necessary for good health and are excellent aids in the elimination of toxins, poisonous acids, and other impurities that accumulate in the system from wrong diet.

Natural fruit acids have an alkaline reaction in the system. The value of a fruit diet for a few days each month cannot be over-estimated, particularly in sickness, chronic ill health, fevers, or any disorder of the system. Germs cannot grow and live in fruit juices. A fruit diet will disinfect the stomach and alimentary canal. Fresh fruits are more effective for this purpose than stewed fruits. Use your fruits fresh, ripe, and uncooked as much as possible. Never sweeten them with refined cane sugar. Use malt sugar, natural sugar, or honey instead.

Fruits are excellent to regulate elimination. They give the body strength and energy. They are natural solvents and should be used extensively in eliminating or reducing diets. Fruit, in fact, is an ideal food. It develops slowly and thus receives the beneficial effects of the sunlight and air for a longer period of time than many other foods.

Fruit juices are the body cleansers and vegetable juices are the body healers; both should be used freely by those seeking to gain or regain health.

Citric, malic, tartaric acids are powerful germicides found in fruits.

Malic acid is found in pineapples, apples, quinces, pears, apricots, plums, peaches, cherries, currants, gooseberries, strawberries, raspberries, blackberries, elderberries, grapes, and tomatoes.

Citric acid is found in strawberries, red raspberries cherries, red currants, cranberries, lemons, limes, grapefruit, and oranges.

Tartaric acid is obtained from grapes and pineapples. Tartaric acid is important in treating all diseases of hyperacidity, such as lung diseases, sore throat, indigestion, etc.

Oxalic acid is found in plums, tomatoes, rhubarb, sorrel, yellow dock, and spinach. It is especially good for constipation and an inactive liver.

Here are some general suggestions on the use of fruit. Do not eat bananas unless they have dark spots on them and the ends are not green. Dried fruits are good if they are not sulphured. Do not mix more than two kinds of fruit at a meal. It is best to eat fruits raw. Applesauce is very good if the whole apple is cooked — skin, core (unless wormy), and seeds — then strain through a colander or sieve. Raisins added to applesauce makes it a very delicate dish.

Foods for Reducing

Before attempting to reduce weight, a cleansing diet of fruits and fruit juices should be taken to rid the body of poisons and excess acids which have been caused by a faulty diet.

Here are some foods that sustain health while reducing:

All fruit juices	All green vegetables
Whole wheat zwieback	Vegetable soups and broths
Cucumbers	Celery
Lettuce	Tomatoes, fresh or canned
Asparagus	Eggplant
Radishes	Watermelon
Cauliflower	Cabbage, raw
Buttermilk	Strawberries
Okra	Turnips
Beets	Beans, fresh string
Peaches	Pineapple (unsweetened)

Fresh fruit or fresh vegetable salads are grand for reducing but do not combine your fruits and vegetables.

Here is a list of "second choice" foods for reducing:

Carrots	Squash	Cranberries
Onions	Oranges	Raspberries

Apricots	Apples	Pears
Parsnips	Lima beans, fresh	Cherries
Grapes	Bananas	Peas, fresh, green
Corn on the cob		

Foods for Gaining Weight

When a person finds it difficult to gain weight it is necessary to cleanse and purify the body with natural, healthful, cleansing foods before trying to build it up. Poisons in the system or an acid prevent proper assimilation. After taking a cleansing diet, use the following foods:

Whole baked potato (sweet and Irish)

Soybean products	Soy cream
Soy mayonnaise	Soy butter
Honey	Protein foods
Oatmeal	Avocados
Coconut	Dates
Whole grain rice	Figs
Soy milk	All nut milks
Oatmeal gruel	Barley gruel
Fruits, sun-dried	Mission figs, sun-dried

Whole grain breads, well-baked
Nuts — almonds, walnuts, pecans

Potatoes, whole grain rice, oatmeal, and soy butter or cream are especially fine for weight-gaining. Eat several raw and also some cooked vegetables daily. Have a glass of orange or pineapple juice at least one-half hour before breakfast — preferably one hour.

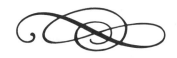

Foods that Supply Minerals

Iron — Spinach, egg yolks, dried peas, dried beans, whole wheat, prunes, watercress, celery, milk, cabbage, oats, lettuce, raisins, apples, English walnuts, lentils, and all greens.

Phosphorus — Legumes, egg yolks, milk, prunes, baked potatoes, nuts, whole cereals, cottage cheese — especially soy cottage cheese.

Calcium — Milk, whole cereals, eggs, cabbage, parsnips, citrus fruits, nuts, legumes, soy milk.

Magnesium — Cherries, apples, nuts, figs, raisins, turnips, prunes, milk, legumes, spinach, whole cereals, soybeans, natural brown rice.

Potassium — Cherries, potatoes, parsnips, turnips, apples, plums, red cabbage, eggplant, cucumbers, soybeans.

Sodium — Strawberries, apples, asparagus, cauliflower, spinach.

Chlorine — Spinach, cabbage, turnips, cauliflower.

Sulphur — Spinach, cabbage, cauliflower, onions, egg yolks.

Lime — Cottage cheese, egg yolk, milk, greens of all kinds, legumes, soybeans.

Fluorine — Cauliflower, cabbage, asparagus, potatoes, spinach.

Silica — Barley, oats, cabbage, onions, oatmeal.

Iodine — Agar-agar, all garden vegetables, beans, peas.

Health-Destroying Foods

Some "foods" could hardly be imagined in the Edenic setting of man's first existence and they are just as alien to his well-being today.

Think, for example, of spices, mustard, pepper, vinegar, salt, condiments, salted meats, canned meats, salted fish, hot sauces, gravies, fried or greasy foods, pastries, very hot or ice-cold foods, cola, all soft drinks, chewing gum, coffee, tea, cocoa, white flour and white-flour products, alcohol, refined sugar and its products.

Such items cannot be compatible with natural Edenic nutritional principles. The organs that make our blood cannot even convert spices, pickles, etc. into pure blood.

Condiments are simply added to make food taste better to a perverted appetite. The taste for condiments is a purely acquired one. Condiments of all kinds are repulsive to infants and to everyone whose taste has not been perverted. They furnish no nutrition and are very irritating to the delicate lining of the stomach and digestive organs. They tend to produce a feverish condition in the system which is very injurious to health and may cause dyspepsia and nervous irritability. Mustard and black pepper cause inflammation of the stomach and skin. Habitual use produces intestinal catarrh and ruins the digestive juices.

The idea that spices and similar substances aid digestion is erroneous. Condiments hinder rather than aid digestion. The oils found in many condiments are irritant and when applied externally in a concentrated form will cause blistering, inflammation, and irritation; and, if the contact is prolonged, will destroy the tissue. The effect upon the stomach is similar. When these poisons are absorbed into the blood they are brought into contact with every cell and fiber of the body. Often the delicate cells of the kidneys undergo a degenerative change from the use of condiments, their efficiency is impaired, and as a result we have Bright's disease and other diseases.

Pickles are indigestible. They resist the action of gastric juice as would pebbles and cause great irritation and chronic diseases. They are hardened by the action of acetic acid and sometimes the addition of alcohol. They arrest the action of saliva and cause gastric catarrh. Acetic acid is an active poison.

Stuffed olives, green olives, brandied fruits, etc., are in the same class. Salads in which vinegar is used are far from wholesome and must always be excluded from the sick or invalid diet — in all cases. Lemon should be substituted for vinegar in all cases. It is an excellent tonic and cleanser for the system.

Free fats can also be injurious and should be used sparingly and then only the best oils with no rancidity — safflower oil, for example. Fats of any kind undergo no change in the stomach. They stay there and resist digestion until they enter the duodenum where the pancreatic juice and bile transform it so it can be absorbed by the system. (Incidentally, the growth-promoting vitamins sometimes associated with fats are bountifully found in greens.)

However, fats are easily digested in the form of nuts, ripe olives, and nut preparations. Nut butter is in every way superior to animal fat and butter and contains no disease germs. (Do not roast the nuts that nut butter is made from.) It is better never to roast nuts because roasting ruins the oil contained in the nut. Good vegetable, nut, and seed oils as used in this book perfectly take the place of all animal fats and butter.

Remember that an excess of fats encourages intestinal putrefaction, biliousness, obesity, congests the liver, promotes heart and arterial diseases, etc.

Also among the injurious "food" products, we must include baking powder. Traditional baking powder contains two chemicals: bicarbonate of soda and tartaric acid. These two chemicals do not neutralize each other in any way so as to render them harmless and there is left in the bread a substance identical with Rochelle salts sold at the drugstore. For an illustration: two teaspoonfuls of baking powder used in a quart of flour leaves in the bread 165 grains of Rochelle salts; that is, 45 grains more than contained in Seidlitz powder. This has no nutritive value but retards digestion and gives the eliminative organs extra work to throw off the poison.

I consider most baking powders on the market to be real poisons. They eat the lining of the stomach or damage it until congestion and inflammation follow. Soda is another injurious substance, decreasing the pancreatic juices that are needed to digest protein, fats, and carbohydrates.

We may almost call cows milk an injurious food. In

my own opinion, cows milk is not suited for human consumption. Half the invalids in the world suffer from dyspepsia and should not take milk. Milk causes constipation, biliousness, coated tongue, and headache and these are the symptoms of intestinal autointoxication. Soy milk and nut milks are excellent substitutes, have practically the same analysis, and do not carry the danger of disease.

Common salt is injurious if used to excess. It should be used very sparingly. It tends to irritate the stomach and blood stream and hinders the digestion of foods. Used to excess, it is one of the causes of rheumatism, dizziness, cancer, scurvy — putting harmful minerals into the system.

Sodium salts are plentifully found in fruits and vegetables such as tomatoes, asparagus, celery, spinach, kale, radishes, turnips, carrots, lettuce, strawberries, and many others.

Salt must not be used in dropsy, hyperacidity, Bright's disease, gastric ulcer, obesity, and epilepsy.

When salt is omitted or reduced, a person soon learns to enjoy the flavors of the food more and he becomes more aware of the infinitely varied and often subtle flavors in natural foods.

Overeating

Even more injurious than many health-destroying foods is the habit of overeating. Overeating or too frequent eating produces a feverish state in the system, overtaxes the digestive organs, the blood becomes impure, and diseases of various kinds occur.

Excessive food also produces excessive acid and causes the gastric mucous membrane to become congested.

An excessive intake of food is much more common than a deficiency. Overfed people are much more likely to have cancer than underfed. Cancer, Bright's disease, arteriosclerosis, high blood pressure, and strokes are some of the consequences of overeating.

It must always be remembered that what would be

enough for a hard-working person would be a great excess for a person of sedentary habits.

The modern method of serving is very destructive. The bill of fare is arranged so that the most highly tempting dishes are presented last, such as pastries, ice cream, etc. This encourages excessive eating. After one has eaten enough, this extra food is added and becomes a poison, a burden to the system.

When the bowels are already full, the second meal is compelled to lie in the stomach overtime and to sour. Overeating increases the work of the stomach, liver, kidneys, and bowels. When this food putrifies, its poisons are absorbed into the blood and the whole system is poisoned.

Food Is Life

Yes, the food question should be given its proper place in the medical world. We are made of what we eat —nothing else — and we should eat to increase strength and preserve health and life. All foods do not agree with everyone, but everyone should eat the natural foods that agree best with him.

Disease and illness would be rare if every bloodstream were pure and if the body were not full of waste matter and toxins.

The human body is a finely constructed machine and transforms energy from the food supplied. As the automobile burns gasoline, the human body burns food. Every machine is consantly wearing and requires renewal of parts; just so, the body must have proper food to build new tissues and to repair worn out ones.

The true science of eating and feeding should be thoroughly understood by all: what elements the system requires in order to build and repair, how best to supply them, and how to prepare them in the most appetizing and life-giving manner.

More information on foods and herbs may be found in **Back To Eden** — the authentic Kloss Family Edition.

Soy Milk
Soy Cheese
Soy Butter and Cream

I have told you some of the amazing nutritional values of soybeans and in later sections you will find recipes for using them in many delicious ways.

Many of these recipes call for various products of soybeans — Soy Milk, Soy Butter, Soy Cream, etc.

Of course, you can buy a good soy milk and always have it on hand, if you prefer; or you can use a good brand of soy milk powder to make up some quickly. But here I want to tell you how to start with the basic ingredients and make, in the least expensive way, these delicious soy products that will perfectly take the place of milk, cream, butter, and even eggs in your cooking — and without some of the harmful qualities of the animal products.

Soy Milk

Soak a pound of soybeans overnight, well covered with water. In the morning wash them thoroughly, remove any broken beans, cover with fresh water, and bring rapidly to a boil. If the water is changed again a couple of times and brought to a boil it helps to remove the "soybean taste" after the milk is made. Then drain the grind while the beans are very hot. Put in a sugar sack, or cheesecloth that is not coarse, and tie the top securely.

Put the sack of ground soybeans in a large dish or pail. Pour 2 quarts of very hot water over them. Knead the sack of ground beans well, washing and squeezing the milk out, then pour off the milk into a large pan or pail. Pour on 2 more quarts of very hot water; knead and squeeze out well again. Combine the second 2 quarts of milk with the first 2 quarts in a large, flat-bottomed pan and boil 20 minutes or more. Stir constantly with a pancake turner from the bottom of the pan until the milk boils; after it is boiling it will not stick to the bottom of the pan.

Sweeten with Malt Honey, honey, or malt sugar. Do not make it too sweet. Salt to taste. Do not cook in aluminum.

Quick Soy Milk

Take 1 pound soy flour (do not have it ground too fine) and 3 quarts of cold water. Mix and boil 25 minutes, strain, sweeten, and salt to taste. It is best to use a flat-bottomed pan and stir with a pancake turner; it burns very easily. If you desire the milk richer add some Soy Cream.

These soy milks may be used in the same way as cows milk. When using for cooking do not sweeten. This milk is wonderfully alkaline. It must be handled in the same way as cows milk. When cooled, keep it in the refrigerator as it will sour in about the same length of time as cows milk. You may add the sweetening to the milk as it is used; it keeps fresh longer before the sweetening is added.

Soy Milk makes a more nourishing and healthful chocolate milk than dairy milk.

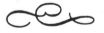

How To Curd Soy Milk

After making the Soy Milk, while the milk is boiling hot, add enough citric acid and it will curd at once. It takes 3 or 4 tablespoons of citric acid to each quart of boiling milk. Stir briskly and let set. The curds form within a few seconds and it isn't long until the milk is curded. Skim the curd off the clear water and place in a double cheesecloth, squeezing out all the water, making the cheese as dry as possible.

If a smooth cheese is desired, use less citric acid. If a granular cheese is liked, use more citric acid.

Soy Buttermilk

Buttermilk is an excellent article of diet for everyday use but is especially beneficial in malnutrition, tuberculosis, toxic conditions, and intestinal infections. Soy Buttermilk has the advantage of producing an alkaline effect and is more nourishing than ordinary buttermilk. It is rich in minerals, very palatable, and more nourishing than yogurt buttermilk used under various names.

Use unsweetened Soy Milk. It may be made of the whole milk or let stand and skim. Let stand until sour as desired or just clabbered and not sour; beat up with an eggbeater and salt to taste.

Soy Butter

Mix together ½ pint water and 2 tablespoons soy flour. Put in a heavy iron frying pan. Boil five minutes, or until thickened. Strain into a mixing bowl. Pour in 1 pint of soy oil, very slowly as in making mayonnaise, beating constantly. (You may use any good oil of your choice.)

Soy Cream

Place in a mixing bowl 1 pint rich Soy Milk and ½ pint soy oil (or any good oil). Pour in the oil in a very small stream, beating constantly until the cream is the desired thickness. If you desire a thick cream use more oil.

If you do not have Soy Milk on hand you can use 1 heaping tablespoon of soy flour and ½ pint of water. Place in a frying pan, stirring with a pancake turner. Let it boil until thickened (five minutes or a little more), then strain and proceed as above, beating in oil until you have the desired thickness.

Soy Cream Cheese

Use unsweetened Soy Milk. Let it stand until it thickens (not sour), put it on the stove and boil a minute or two until the water separates from the whey. Put it into cheesecloth and wring dry. Run through the grinder used in making the milk until you have a smooth paste. Add a little rich Soy Milk to soften and make a creamy consistency. Salt to taste. Soy Mayonnaise may also be added with advantage.

Soy Cottage Cheese

Make in the same way as ordinary cottage cheese. Allow the milk to sour or clabber, then heat to body temperature until the curd separates from the whey. Drain in a very fine sieve or through cheesecloth. When it has drained dry add a little rich Soy Milk to soften and flavor, as you would add cream to ordinary cottage cheese. The addition of a little Soy Mayonnaise improves the flavor; makes a richer product. Salt to taste. You may add a little honey to make a tasty spread for children — a splendid nerve builder. Use unsweetened Soy Milk.

Soy Cheese

Thoroughly mix 5 pounds of raw peanut butter with the 1 quart of tomato purée (you may use 2 quarts tomato puree if you prefer a strong tomato flavor). Stir in gradually 5 quarts Soy Milk and put in a warm place until it develops lactic acid or until it gets about as sour as sour cottage cheese.

After the cheese has developed lactic acid enough and is as sour as you like, put it in tin cans (either No. 2 or No. 3), seal with a home can sealer and place in a large vessel (an old-fashioned wash boiler or kettle) and cover with boiling water. Let cook for four or five hours, keeping the cans covered with boiling water. If you have a steam pressure cooker, keep the cans under five pounds pressure for four hours. The cheese is then ready to be opened and served.

You can make up a smaller amount and cook in a double boiler for about 2 hours, then let cool and serve.

Quick Soy Cheese

> 1 cup soy flour   3 cups water
> Juice of 2 lemons

Bring the water to a boil in a saucepan. Mix the soy flour to a paste with cold water. Beat for a minute with an egg beater and add to boiling water. Cook about five minutes. Add the lemon juice, then set aside to cool. Strain the curds through a fine strainer or cheesecloth.

This cheese is an excellent base for patties, loaves, and other entrées. It may also be pressure cooked for an hour (10 pounds pressure) and then served cold in salads or other dishes.

Original Soy Cheese

> 1 cup dry soy beans (Yellow   Juice of 2 lemons
>   Mammoth are good)

Soak beans overnight, drain off liquid, and wash well. Remove any broken pieces. Use ½ cup beans at a time to 1 cup very hot water and run in a liquefier for two to three minutes. (Hold a lid over the liquefier to avoid splashing the hot water.) Strain the milk through a fine sieve.
Put all the pulp back in the liquefier, nearly covered with liquid. Liquefy for about two minutes and strain again into the soy milk.

To make milk into soy cheese, bring to a good boil (a double boiler will help prevent sticking). Add the lemon juice, stirring enough to mix well.

Allow to stand in a warm place until the mixture is coagulated. Then strain through a fine cheesecloth.

This soy cheese may be used in patties, loaves, or other entrees.

If used in salads or in other dishes that are not cooked, pressure cook cheese for an hour (10 pounds pressure) and let cool.

A Substitute for Egg Yolk

You may use the following in any recipe where it is desired to use the yolk of an egg. This product looks very much like egg yolk, tastes like it, and has very much the same properties.

Take 1 heaping tablespoon of soy flour, mix with ½ cup of water, put in a frying pan and boil until it thickens, stirring constantly so it does not stick. Strain into a mixing bowl and beat in soy oil until it becomes thick enough to be cut with a knife.

Use this wherever the yolk of egg is desired. Season with a pinch of salt and use dandelion butter coloring, if you wish, for a little added color.

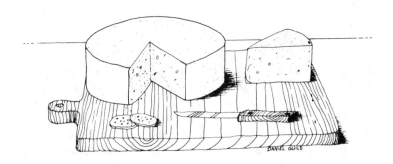

Nut Milk
Nut Cheese
Nut Butter and Cream

Nut Milk

1 cup raw peanut butter
$\frac{1}{2}$ cup Milk Sweetening
  (see recipe)

1 cup boiling water
Few grains of salt

Mix the peanut butter and the Milk Sweetening thoroughly together. Use 1 heaping teaspoon of this mixture to 1 cup of boiling water. Thoroughly mix, adding salt.

This may be used as any other milk.

Nut Cheese

1 pound raw peanut butter
$1\frac{1}{2}$ pints water or Soy Milk

$\frac{1}{2}$ pound Soy Butter
Salt to taste

Pour the water into the peanut butter very slowly, stirring to a paste, gradually adding water until the entire amount has been used. If Soy Milk is used instead of water, a better product is obtained. Let stand until it sours to suit the taste, thus developing lactic acid like the lactic acid in buttermilk. Beat in the Soy Butter. Put in cans, seal them with a home can sealer, and place in a vessel to cook for four or more hours as directed for cooking Soy Cheese.

If you have a pressure cooker, the canned cheese should be cooked under five or six pounds of pressure for four hours.

You may also cook this in a double boiler for about two hours, then cool and serve.

Dieter's Nut Cheese

1 pound raw peanut butter	1½ pints water
4 tablespoons ground oatmeal flour	Salt to taste

Prepare in the same manner as directed for Nut Cheese (above).

Some of the nut cheeses I make are much like the yellow American cheese and others are similar to cream cheese. They are very agreeable to the taste, and are high in food value. Emulsified nut oils are much easier to digest and contain none of the harmful bacteria of ordinary cheeses. These nut cheeses may be put up in cans to keep them pure and sanitary. They are prepared in a way that develops lactic acid such as is found in yogurt buttermilk and cottage cheese.

Those who cannot eat ordinary cheese made with rennet can eat freely of Nut Cheese and there is no exposure to disease as is the case with other cheeses.

Nut Cheese is more economical and may be used in any way that the cheeses on the market are used. More food value is obtained for the money.

Malted Nut Cream

1 pound raw peanut butter	¼ pound Malt Honey
2 ounces malt powder	(see recipe)

Mix the ingredients together and put up in cans. It will keep indefinitely.

Superb Peanut Butter

1 pound blanched raw
   peanuts (see below)
1 pound coconut oil

Butter coloring
Salt to taste

Boil peanuts until they are done but not enough to make tham fall to pieces. Do not use too much water. Run the peanuts and coconut oil through a peanut butter mill; add salt and a very little dandelion butter coloring. This is an excellent and wholesome butter. Peanut butter made this way can be diluted with water and used as cream or spread on bread.

Blanched Peanut Butter

Cover one pound blanched peanuts (see below) with water. Boil until they just begin to become tender but not mushy. Drain off the water and dry the peanuts thoroughly. This can be done in the sun, or in a very slow oven if they are stirred frequently, but the nuts must not be browned at all. Grind them fine.

This makes an excellent butter which can be used in many ways. Add water until it is of the consistency of milk or cream to eat with vegetables or fruit. This same butter may be reduced with water, beaten in coconut oil with butter coloring added, and salted to taste, making a palatable and nourishing butter which is easy to digest.

Simple Nut Butter

Select any amount of fresh nuts. Grind them through the very finest disc or nut butter grinder.

To Blanch Peanuts

Buy shelled nuts and heat slightly. Do not heat too much; only until they are a very light, golden brown. Just heat so they are slightly dextrinized. Rub between the hands or place on a table and lightly press with a rolling pin to loosen the skins sufficiently to enable one to blow them away.

Nut Meal

Made like nut butter except that the second-to-finest grinding disc is used.

Nut Butter Cream

Gradually add warm water to nut butter to make a smooth paste. Warm water can be added until the paste is of the creamy consistency desired.

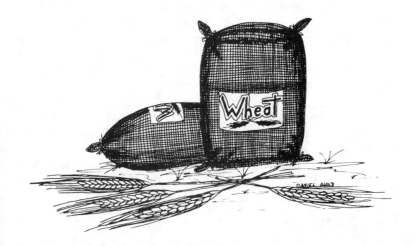

Main Dishes

Main dishes without meat or animal products, without refined products, very high in protein and general nutritional value and with good eye and taste appeal: these are the objectives of this important section of **The Back To Eden Cookbook.**

Basic Wheat Protein

Wheat gluten alone is not a well-balanced protein food. It must be combined with other vegetable proteins. It does lend a meaty texture to roasts, loaves, and other main dishes and thus is a useful product — just remember its nutritional limitations.

To make a basic wheat gluten, take 5 pounds of strong gluten flour, ordinarily called "bread flour." It can be obtained at health food stores, mills, bakeries, or major grocers.) Add 2 quarts of water and make a fairly stiff dough, about the consistency of bread dough. Let stand for an hour after mixing. Then put into a large pan and cover with water. Wash out the starch by working it with both hands. When the water becomes white with starch, pour it off and put in fresh water. Repeat this until the water is clear; then all the starch will be washed out.

If it is desired to have the gluten very tender, cover it with water and let stand a day or two under water. If the weather is cool it should stand about two days but in warm weather a day will be sufficient time. Do not let it stand too long, however, for the gluten will dissolve.

Then cut the gluten mass into small pieces, dropping them as cut into a pan of boiling water — enough water so that the gluten will float. Stir with a pancake turner on the bottom so it will not burn. Let cook for half an hour.

Remove from the water what is desired for immediate use and add a little soy sauce for a meaty flavor. Always keep the gluten covered with water, both before it is cooked and afterwards.

It can be warmed in a frying pan with a little oil and seasoned with finely cut onions if desired. Too much frying makes it tough, however.

This wheat protein can be used in stews, potpies, vegetable roasts, or any place where lean beefsteak is used. It is excellent in vegetable soup.

Peanut Gluten Roast

8 ounces strong Cereal Coffee (see recipe)	5 ounces raw peanut meal
	Salt to taste
1 pound washed gluten	

This makes a better protein balance than the gluten alone. Run this mixture through an Enterprise mill two or three times. Put it into cans, seal, and cook in a steam pressure cooker for about four hours under five pounds of pressure; or if in an open kettle, for six hours. The roast can also be put into a stone crock (with the crock placed in a dish of water) and baked four hours in a moderate oven. The dish of water is to prevent the roast from burning. It can also be baked in a tin can (cover with foil).

This product will be found to be an excellent product when cut into cubes to combine with any kind of a vegetable stew that the housewife may wish to prepare.

Protein Patties

2 cups ground gluten	1/2 cup soy sauce
2 cups cooked brown rice	1/2 teaspoon salt
1 onion, finely chopped	

Flavor with garlic, sage, or Savory Seasoning. Mix thoroughly, make into patties, and brown in oven or frying pan.

Vegetable Sauerbraten with Noodles

2 cups ground cooked gluten	1 teaspoon salt
2 onions chopped fine	2 tablespoons brown sugar
4 tablespoons oil	1/2 cup chopped celery
2 tablespoons flour	1 bay leaf
2/3 cup lemon juice	1/2 teaspoon celery salt
2 cups water	1/3 cup soy sauce

Combine all ingredients except gluten and cook into a sauce. Rub the sauce through a sieve and pour over gluten. Bake in a covered casserole for one hour.

Vegetable Potpie

2 cups gluten pieces	2 tablespoons oil
2 large potatoes	1 teaspoon Savory Seasoning
1 onion	(see recipe)
1 or 2 carrots	2 cups water
2 stalks celery	1 teaspoon salt
2 tablespoons flour	

Dice the potatoes and other vegetables, add salt and enough water to cover. Cook in an open kettle until water has evaporated. Coat gluten pieces with seasoned corn meal, brown in oil, then cut up into one-inch bits. Combine flour and oil in a heated pan, add Savory Seasoning and water. Salt to taste. Mix all ingredients, put in casserole and cover with piecrust. Brown in hot oven.

Vegetable Salmon

1 pound raw peanut butter	1 No. 2 can of tomatoes
1 medium-sized carrot,	put through a fine sieve
finely ground or grated	1 pint water

Mix ingredients thoroughly, salt to taste. Put into cans, if desired, seal and cook under five pounds steam pressure for four hours. If cooked in an ordinary kettle, well-covered with water, it will require one and a half to two hours more.

The mixture can also be baked in the oven. First, boil it a few minutes in an open saucepan, stirring constantly until it thickens; then bake in a slow oven for an hour. It is then ready to serve.

It may also be cooked in a double boiler for about three hours. Put into a pan and slice when cold. This is a very wholesome and palatable dish.

Light and Delightful Peanut Butter Loaf

½ cup water	1 tablespoon cornstarch
6 tablespoons peanut butter	or other thickener
1 cup tomato juice	2 tablespoons minced onion
1 cup (or more) dried	Salt and sage to taste
bread crumbs	

Mix peanut butter thoroughly with water. Add other ingredients and steam two hours in double boiler. It may then be packed in a loaf pan and cooled for slicing. Mix with Soy Mayonnaise for sandwich spread.

Soybean Loaf

2 cups soybeans,	1⅓ cups whole wheat
cooked and ground	zwieback crumbs
2 cups pinto bean pulp	1 onion, chopped fine
1 cup tomato juice	2 tablespoons soy sauce
1 cup finely chopped nuts	Salt to taste

Mix ingredients thoroughly. Add sage, celery seed, thyme, or other flavoring as you like, put in oiled baking dish and bake one hour in moderate oven.

Soy Cottage Cheese Loaf

3 cups Soy Cottage Cheese
  (see recipe)
³/₄ cup raw peanut butter
1 cup whole wheat bread
  crumbs, toasted
¹/₄ cup peanut oil
6 tablespoons lemon juice
6 tablespoons soy sauce

1 tablespoon chopped garlic
1 heaping teaspoon sage
Pinch cayenne pepper
¹/₂ cup celery, chopped
Parsley
1 cup chopped onion
¹/₂ cup chopped green pepper
Salt to taste

Chop the celery, parsley, onion, and pepper very fine. Mix with the lemon juice, soy sauce, peanut butter, and Soy Cottage Cheese. Add other ingredients, mix thoroughly, and bake in a moderate oven.

German Cabbage Beroks

2 cups ground gluten
2 pounds bread dough
  (see recipe)
3 onions, chopped fine

¹/₂ large cabbage,
  chopped fine
Seasonings of your choice

Wilt chopped cabbage and onions in heated, oiled skillet. Add ground gluten and seasonings. Roll out dough and cut into thin, three-inch squares. Place spoonful of filling on each dough square, fold over and pinch edges together — use a fork. Place squares upside down on oiled baking sheet. Let rise, and bake in moderate oven.

Italian Meat Balls

2 cups vegetable loaf of
  your choice (see recipes)
1 cup cracker crumbs
¹/₂ cup whole wheat flour
¹/₂ cup Soy Milk (see recipe)
¹/₄ cup tomato juice

1¹/₂ teaspoons Savory
  Seasoning (see recipe)
²/₃ cup bread crumbs
¹/₂ cup onion, minced
Sage and celery seasoning
Salt to taste

Mix all the ingredients and form into croquettes. Bake in an oiled pan. Serve with tomato sauce.

Nature's Own Meat Loaf

2 cups raw peanut butter
¹/₂ cup boiled kidney beans
2 tablespoons ground onions

3 cups water
Ground celery seed to taste

Mix the ingredients, put in can, seal with a home can sealer, and cook for four hours under five pounds pressure. The roast can also be placed in a crock and baked in the oven, using a flat pan of water to prevent burning as in recipe below. May be baked in tin cans (covered with foil).

This roast can be used diced in roasts, stews, and soups. It is good sliced and browned for sandwiches.

Peanut Roast

1 pound raw peanut butter
1¹/₂ pints water

Salt to taste

Add water slowly to peanut butter, stirring continuously to make paste free from lumps. Boil from one to four hours.

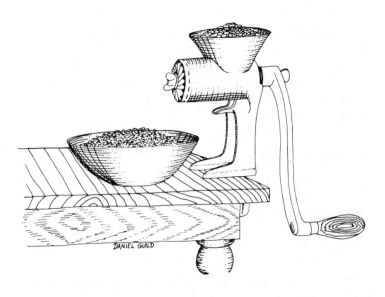

DANIEL GUILD

Can be boiled in a double boiler or cooked in the oven by placing the dish containing the roast in a dish of water to prevent it from burning on bottom and sides. May also be cooked in cans as in the recipe above.

The roast should be of such a consistency that, when cold, it can be sliced and eaten. Children and people with delicate digestions may eat this roast. It is good in sandwiches; also diced in roasts or in stews and soups.

Tomato Loaf

Make this loaf just like Peanut Roast but use half water and half tomato juice; or you can use all tomato juice if you like.

Scotch Barley Roast

1³/₄ cups pearl barley	1 cup water
4 cups Savory Broth	2 medium onions, chopped
(see recipes)	¹/₂ cup toasted almonds
1 cup oil	¹/₂ pound sharp Soy Cheese
2 4-ounce cans mushrooms	(see recipe)

Brown barley in oil. Sauté almonds, mushrooms, onions, and add to barley.

Pour in 2 cups broth and put in covered casserole. Bake 45 minutes in moderate oven.

Add 2 more cups of broth and bake another 45 minutes. Stir in the last cup of liquid mixed with the Soy Cheese. Bake 30 minutes more and sprinkle top with a little grated Soy Cheese.

Lentil-Potato Roast

2 cups cooked lentils	1 chopped onion
1 cup cooked potatoes, diced	1 tablespoon Savory Sauce
1 4-ounce can sliced	(see recipe)
mushrooms	2 tablespoons flour
¹/₄ tablespoon salt	2 cups Soy Milk (see recipe)
4 tablespoons oil	

Sauté onions and mushrooms in margarine; add savory sauce and flour, then milk, and cook a few minutes. Add lentils and cook a few minutes more. Pour over diced potatoes and mix well. Put in casserole and sprinkle with oil. Bake until thoroughly hot.

Savory Soy Loaf

1 pound Soy Cheese	1 tablespoon lemon juice
2 cups tomato juice	1½ teaspoon Soy Butter
¼ cup Savory Broth	2 teaspoons grated onion
(see recipes)	1 bay leaf
½ tablespoon sage	1 tablespoon chopped parsley
1 tablespoon celery salt	1 tablespoon Savory Seasoning
1 tablespoon flour	

Combine all ingredients and bake one-half hour in loaf pan.

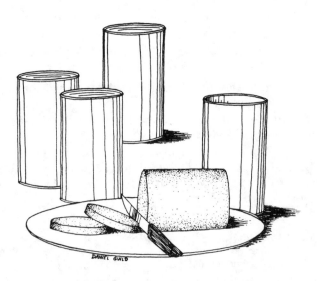

Golden Nut Loaf

2 cups ground carrots	5 cups wheat crackers,
1 cup ground nuts, any kind	crushed
1 cup cooked rice	1 teaspoon sage
2 cups dry bread crumbs	2 tablespoons Soy Cream
$^1/_2$ cup chopped onions	Salt, celery salt, to taste

Cook carrots until tender, grind them and add rice and crushed wheat crackers. Soak the bread crumbs until soft, squeeze out the water and measure out 2 cups of crumbs. Mix all ingredients and bake in oiled loaf pan. Brush some oil on the top of loaf before baking and sprinkle with cracker crumbs. Bake until done and serve with tomato sauce.

Vegetable Hash

2 potatoes	2 large onions
1 carrot	$^1/_2$ cup peas
3 stalks celery	1 teaspoon chopped parsley
2 cups tomato pulp	$^1/_2$ teaspoon sage
$^1/_2$ No. 2 can corn	$^1/_2$ teaspoon thyme
$^1/_2$ cup cut string beans	

Finely dice potatoes, carrots, onions and celery. Cook until tender and pour into colander to drain. Mix all ingredients, then add tomatoes, parsley, and herbs. Salt to taste. Add a sauce (see recipes) and bake 30-40 minutes.

Flavorful Nut and Potato Hash

3 cups diced cold boiled	3 tablespoons diced onion
potatoes	2 tablespoons oil
1$^1/_2$ cups diced cold Peanut	$^1/_4$ teaspoon sage or marjoram
Roast (see recipe)	2 tablespoons brown flour
or other nut loaf	$^1/_2$ cup water
$^1/_2$ cup Soy Milk	Salt to taste

Heat the oil, onion, and herbs in a small saucepan for a few minutes but do not brown. Add browned flour, then a small quantity of the Soy Milk, and stir until smooth. Add remainder of milk and water and boil. Salt to taste and add the diced Peanut Roast to the gravy. Lightly salt the diced potatoes, then pour the hot mixture over them and mix. Put into an oiled pan, sprinkle with a little Soy Milk or oil and bake to a light brown.

Seasoned Lentil "Cutlets"

2 cups cooked lentils, well-drained, firm	2 cups mashed potatoes with seasonings of your choice
3 tablespoons chopped onion	1/2 teaspoon sage or
2 tablespoons Soy Butter	sweet marjoram

Combine onion, seasonings, and Soy Butter into a small pan and simmer briefly to soften the onion. Do not brown. Add the lentils and mix with the potato. Form into small patties and brown lightly in a hot oven or oiled skillet.

Lentil and Rice Loaf

1 cup lentil purée	3 tablespoons Soy Milk
2 cups steamed rice	Sprinkle of sage
1 tablespoon chopped onion	1/3 cup chopped walnuts
1 tablespoon oil	Salt to taste
1 tablespoon browned flour	

Put the butter, onion, and seasoning into a small saucepan and simmer for a few minutes. Add the browned flour, then the milk, and stir until smooth. Salt to taste. Mix in the rice with a fork. Combine all ingredients, pack lightly in an oiled bread tin, and bake until hot through and slightly browned on top.

Soy Patties

2 cups soybean pulp	1 onion chopped fine
2 cups cooked natural brown rice	1 tablespoon soy sauce
	1/2 teaspoon salt
2 tablespoons oil	Garlic or sage

Mix ingredients thoroughly, make into patties, roll in whole wheat bread crumbs and bake in greased pan until brown, or warm in a frying pan — but do not fry.

Nutty Lentil-Rice Loaf

3 cups steamed rice	1/4 cup Soy Milk
1 1/3 cups cooked lentils	1/4 teaspoon sage
(soft or puréed)	1/3 cup chopped walnuts
1 tablespoon chopped onion	Salt to taste
1 tablespoon browned flour	

Simmer onion in a small amount of oil for a few minutes. Add milk to browned flour and stir until smooth. Add seasoning. Add remaining ingredients and place in oiled baking dish. Bake until hot and slightly browned on top.

Nut Loaf Orient

2 cups cooked brown rice	2 tablespoons chopped onions
1 cup nuts, chopped	2 tablespoons chopped celery
1/2 cup whole wheat bread	Salt to taste
crumbs, toasted	Soy Milk to moisten
2 tablespoons soy sauce	

Chop onions and celery fine, mix all ingredients together, add more Soy Milk if too dry and bake in moderate oven 45 minutes.

Italian Baked Rice

1 cup uncooked brown rice	2 tablespoons oil
1/2 cup macaroni pieces	A sprinkle of thyme
2 tablespoons chopped onion	1 1/2 cups tomato pulp
1 small clove garlic	2 1/2 cups water
2 tablespoons diced green	Salt
pepper	

Heat the rice in a frying pan or in a hot oven, stirring often, until light brown in color. Add 1/4 teaspoon salt and the water. Cook in a covered saucepan until dry. Cook the macaroni in boiling, salted water until done; then wash and drain. Put green pepper, onion, garlic, and thyme into a saucepan with the oil, and stir briefly over heat.

Add the tomato, salt to taste, bring to a boil and pour over the rice. Mix well. Put a layer of the rice-tomato in an oiled baking pan and sprinkle the cooked macaroni over it. Pour the remainder of the rice mixture over the macaroni; bake in a medium oven 30 minutes.

Seasoned Rice-Nut Patties

2 cups cooked rice	4 tablespoons chopped onion
1 cup zwieback crumbs	1 tablespoon oil
3/4 cup Soy Milk	1 cup chopped walnuts
1/2 teaspoon sage or marjoram	Salt

Simmer onion, seasonings, and oil in a small pan. Add milk and a 1/4 teaspoon salt. Bring to a boil, then pour over the crumbs. Let stand 10 minutes. Add nuts; mix in the steamed rice. Form into small patties and brown.

Southern Nut-Rice Loaf

2 cups cooked brown rice	1 tablespoon finely chopped onion
1 cup peanut butter (diluted to consistency of thin cream)	1 teaspoon sage
	Salt to taste

Mix together (mixture should be thin) and bake in a moderate oven 20 to 30 minutes.

Parsleyed Rice Meat Balls

1/4 cup Soy Milk or tomato juice	1 chopped onion, small
1 cup whole grain bread crumbs	1/2 teaspoon celery salt
2 tablespoons fresh parsley	1/2 teaspoon salt
	1/4 cup unbleached flour
	2 cups cooked rice

Mix all ingredients (saving aside a cup of the bread crumbs). Roll in oiled baking pan until lightly coated with oil. Sprinkle crumbs on loaf and bake in moderate oven until golden brown. May be served with hot tomato sauce.

Old-Fashioned Spanish Rice

½ cup natural rice
2½ tablespoons oil
2 tablespoons diced green
    pepper
1½ cups hot water

1½ tablespoons slightly
    browned flour
1½ cups tomato pulp
3 tablespoons diced onion
Sprinkle of sage

Brown the rice in a frying pan or in a hot oven until a very light brown. Add the hot water and let boil gently until the water is evaporated and the rice looks dry. Cover and let stand for 10 minutes. Put the oil, onion, green pepper, and seasonings into a small pan and simmer a few minutes. Add the flour, then a little of the tomato, and stir smooth. Add the rest of the tomato and boil 5 minutes. Salt to taste and pour over the cooked rice. Mix well and steam until of a consistency to dish up nicely.

Jerusalem Fillets

1 dozen chopped ripe olives
2 tablespoons chopped onion
2 teaspoons chopped parsley
2 tablespoons whole wheat
    flour

⅓ cup Soy Milk
Sage or marjoram
Salt to taste
1 tablespoon oil

Simmer butter, onion, parsley, and seasonings in a small saucepan for a few minutes. Add the flour and chopped olives and mix. Add milk and blend until smooth. Cut bread into thin slices, trim off crusts, and oil very lightly. Cover with a spread of the olive mixture and cover that with another slice of bread. Press together and cut into triangles. Place in an oiled baking pan, pour over it a thin cream-tomato sauce and let simmer in the oven until hot.

Vegetable Tamale

12 ears corn (1 large can of corn may be used)	1 onion
4 cups water	1 teaspoon oil
1 No. 2½ can tomatoes	1 teaspoon salt

Cut the corn from cobs, then scrape the cobs and wash with the water in order to save the juice. Combine corn with the liquid and put through a sieve. Add other ingredients, salt lightly, and cook briefly in oven. Stir well before serving.

Baking Or Canning Beans

Use any kind of beans. Soak overnight in cold water, then mix with tomato sauce or other seasoning if you prefer, and bake in a stone jar about four hours in a hot oven. One who cannot eat beans prepared in the ordinary way can eat them baked in this fashion.

The same beans, after soaking overnight, may also be put up in cans. (Fill the cans about three-fourths full, then fill to the top with salted water. Or use half tomato sauce and half water.) Seal in a home can sealer and cook in a steam pressure cooker, using 10 pounds pressure for about an hour and a half. Some beans require a little less cooking and some a little more. Test them for yourself. Old beans require longer cooking than new ones but all beans should be thoroughly soft and tender. Prepared properly, they will not produce gas and will digest more easily.

Another way to prepare beans is to cook them until almost dry, then put them in a pan or some kind of a dish, add some Soy Milk, put in the oven, and bake thoroughly.

Sprouted Soybeans

Soak the beans overnight. Pour the water off, put the beans in a warm place, rinsing several times a day for several days. Let them sprout about half an inch. Parboil for four or five minutes. Pour the water off, then put the beans into any kind of a cooking vessel and let boil until tender. A little tomato and onion makes a very palatable and wholesome dish.

They are much better if cooked in a steam pressure cooker for about 40 minutes or more. Some beans require more and some less cooking, depending on the variety.

Seasoned Soy Beans

1 quart soy beans	1 onion
2 teaspoons salt	1 large bay leaf
1/4 cup sugar	1/2 teaspoon thyme
1 1/2 cups tomato purée	1/4 cup oil

Soak the beans overnight. Pour off the water and add remaining ingredients and water enough to cover beans. Cook for three hours in a pressure cooker at a pressure of ten pounds.

Southern Style Soy Beans

2 cups cooked soybeans	1/2 cup bread crumbs
2 cups tomatoes	2 teaspoons salt
2 cups corn	

Alternate layers of beans, corn, and strained tomatoes in an oiled baking dish. Pour the salted juice drained from tomatoes over the mixture. Cover with bread crumbs and bake in a moderate oven 30 minutes, or until crumbs are browned.

Boston Baked Beans

1 cup navy beans	1 tablespoon sorghum or
1 teaspoon salt	maple syrup, or honey

Soak the beans overnight. Gradually heat to boiling, then add seasoning. Place in a bean crock and cover with water.

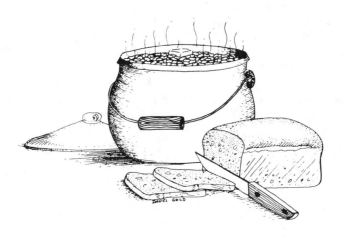

Bake in slow oven 6 to 12 hours. Keep the beans below boiling point and see that they are always covered with liquid. Lentils may be baked in the same way.

Raw Spinach Sandwich

Chop enough raw spinach to fill one cup. Salt and mix with Soy Mayonnaise. You may also add finely chopped celery and onion.

Toasted Tomato Sandwich

Put slices of ripe tomato between slices of whole wheat bread spread with Soy Mayonnaise or Soy Butter. Put on cookie sheet and toast in oven. Serve warm.

Using Sprouted Seeds

Since before the turn of the century it has been a part of the Kloss health program to advocate the use of sprouted grains and legumes for enhanced nutritional value.

Sprouting seeds, of course, is far from new. It has been done in many lands from the earliest times.

The sprouting of any bean, pea, or grain turns the protein to a great extent, into peptones, simple amino acids, and the starch into dextrose or maltose for greater digestibility and energy. The sprouts are very high in vitamins — more so even than spinach, lettuce, or celery — as well as other life-giving elements.

Almost any seed can be successfully sprouted and used in salads, breads, loafs, and sandwiches or eaten plain.

Place in a large jar a couple of tablespoons of smaller seeds. Cover well with water and let stand overnight. Pour off water. Rewash two or three times daily, pouring off water, and keeping the jar in a dark place for approximately three days or until the seeds are well-sprouted.

Allow to stand until the sprouts are about one-half inch long. The time will vary somewhat. Lentils, for example, do not take as long as soybeans. Soybeans may be allowed to sprout until they are an inch long and then only the sprouts eaten, if you wish.

Sprouts alone need only a few minutes cooking. Most sprouts may be eaten raw and with or without the seeds. Cook sprouted seeds in any way you would cook them unsprouted — remembering that the sprouted seeds do not require as much cooking because they are already somewhat "predigested."

You will discover ways of rubbing and floating away the tough husks left from seeds although they will not harm a normal digestive system.

Sprouted Lentil Roast

2 cups gluten pieces (see recipe)

2 cups sprouted lentils

Mix together and run through a grinder two or three times. Season with a little tomato and sage. Salt to taste. Cook four hours in sealed tins under five pounds pressure. If tins are "canned" in an open vessel or double boiler, six hours cooking is required.

To cook in the oven, make the material into a loaf and cover with water — not too much. Place this dish in another containing water and bake. (This is to prevent burning.) When done, pour the liquid off the loaf and use for a gravy. It may be thickened with corn meal and seasoned with a savory seasoning of your choice.

Sprouted Soybeans with Rice

Boil the sprouted soybeans until tender. Boil unpolished rice separately. Mix approximately equal parts, add tomato sauce and some cubes of Nut Meal. Mix all together and place in the oven. Bake slowly, leaving uncovered the last few minutes to brown the top.

If the flavor of the soybeans is too strong, they may be parboiled in strong salt water for a few minutes before mixing with the rice. Be sure to wash them thoroughly after parboiling.

Soybean Sprout Salad

Let soybean grow until two inches long. Chop the sprouts with equal amounts of celery, cabbage, or lettuce. Add some chopped olives and tomato. Season with lemon juice and salt or any desired dressing.

Mung bean sprouts or any other sprout may be used in this salad. Try a combination of sprouts if you wish.

Vegetarian Chop Suey

1 cup lightly cooked mung bean or soybean sprouts	1 onion
½ cup cooked mushrooms	1 tablespoon soy sauce
½ cup celery	½ cup vegetarian loaf of your choice (see recipes)

Chop the mushrooms and onion and brown lightly. Cut celery in short strips and cook until just tender. Dice and add vegetarian loaf.

Mix all ingredients, season with salt and soy sauce. If

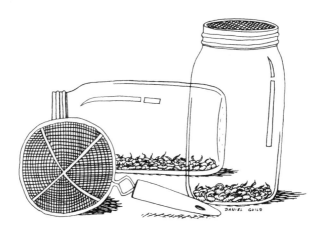

necessary add a little water and heat for 10 minutes. Serve with cooked brown rice (see recipes).

If such things as water chestnuts and bamboo shoots are available they make interesting additions to this simple recipe.

Sprout Sandwich

A delightful, savory open-faced sandwich may be made by putting Soy Butter or Soy Mayonnaise on a piece of warm, whole wheat bread, laying on a generous amounts of sprouts (smaller ones like alfalfa sprouts) and sprinkling with brewer's yeast.

Bread
...a Health Food

Bread is not only a "health food"; it is the most important one. "There is more religion in a loaf of good bread than many think," Ellen G. White once said. Properly baked bread made from the right material — whole grain flours — has been the staff of life from earliest history and is one of the principal foods God gave to man.

How sad that it has been made the "staff of death" by the modern inventions of milling and baking. God never intended that wheat and other grains should be separated into different parts, presented as a wonderful invention and sold for a big price. Refined flour is indeed an invention to destroy both soul and body. Untold harm is done by many baked goods found on the market today.

However, it is possible to live as we were intended to live — on whole wheat bread, whole rye bread, or whole barley bread, with vegetables or fruit added.

Even oats make an excellent bread. An especially delicious bread can be made by taking part whole wheat flour, whole corn flour, whole oats flour, and whole soybean flour. Add a little Malt Honey or natural syrup. This will make a bread that anyone can live and work on by eating just a little fruit with it.

Before grains are ripe, in the milky state, all of them can be eaten raw. They are then in the grape-sugar state — like the sugar found in thoroughly ripe fruit. After the grain ripens, the sugar turns to starch; and the human system has no fluid to digest raw starch properly to make good blood. Animals have different fluids than man and can digest raw starch.

The baking process has an effect on this starch very similar to the ripening of fruit on a tree. There, the sun and the air gradually change the fruit starch to grape sugar. When bread is put into the oven it goes through a similar process. The prolonged baking gradually changes the starch, to a large extent, into grape sugar; thus making it fit for digestion. In other words, it puts it into a form on which the digestive fluids can properly act to make good blood.

According to the ancient record, the baking process was instituted by God Himself in order to prepare the grains and starchy foods so they could be eaten by man and properly nourish him.

(Most commercial baked goods are baked just enough to stand up but not enough to kill the yeast germ; nor are they baked enough to change the starch so it can be easily digested.)

Grains and Legumes for Better Protein

In Bible times they used to combine various grains and legumes for bread making. For example, note this instruction in Ezekiel 4:9: "Take thou also unto thee wheat, and barley, and beans, and lentils, and millet and fitches, and put them in one vessel, and make the bread thereof . . ."

We know today that a combination of grains and legumes provides a more complete protein than any one of these foods alone.

A number of seeds have also been used in bread since Abraham's time: caraway, gimmel, annise, rue, fennel, dill, and sesame. All of these have medicinal properties. They all are good for indigestion and they prevent fermentation. For gas and colic, rue was quite frequently used; it was used even by the priests in Christ's time. It has a wonderfully-quiet, soothing effect upon tired and weary nervous systems.

People would do well today if they would use more of these things instead of the abundant luxuries that destroy both soul and body.

Breads are of two kinds: fermented and unfermented. Fermented bread is made light by a ferment; yeast usually being employed. Unfermented bread is made light by the introduction of air into the dough or batter. This method will be described later.

Yeast or Fermented Bread

Fermented bread is generally made by mixing flour, water, salt, and yeast into a dough. A small amount of malt extract, Malt Honey, or honey may be added if desired, for it increases the food value and hastens fermentation. This is the straight dough method.

This dough is kneaded until it is elastic to the touch and does not stick to the board, the object being to incorporate air and to distribute the yeast uniformly. The dough is then covered and allowed to rise until it has doubled its bulk and does not respond to the touch when tapped sharply; but rather, gradually and stubbornly begins to sink.

At this stage, the dough is "ripe" and ready to be worked down. It will require from two to three and a half hours to rise to this point depending on the grade and consistency of the flour used, the temperature of the room in which it is set, and the amount of yeast used. This process is best accomplished at a temperature ranging from 80 to 90 degrees. The bread is again worked down well, turned over in the bowl, and left to rise until about three-fourths its original bulk. Then it is turned out on a board, worked enough to expel the air, and cut up in the size pieces desired for a loaf. (An ordinary pound loaf requires a pound plus three or four ounces of dough.)

Mold the pieces until the air has been worked out and leave them on the board a few minutes so they will rise just a little. You will find that this improves the texture of the bread. Then form the pieces into loaves and knead enough to work out the air. Do not knead too much. With a little experience you will become a master at bread making.

Unleavened Bread

Unfermented or unleavened bread is made light by the introduction of air into the dough or batter. This is done by means of beating batter breads or kneading dough breads.

Sponge Bread

Bread is also made by setting a "sponge" at the beginning by making a batter of the water, yeast, and part of the flour; letting it rise until it is light, then adding the remaining ingredients and working all into a dough. This is called the sponge method. Bun and cracker dough is usually set with a sponge, as they require a very fine and light texture, best obtained by this method. A sponge is light enough when it appears frothy and full of bubbles. The time required will vary with the quantity and quality of yeast used and with the temperature of the room in which it is set to rise.

Yeast

A very convenient yeast is compressed cake yeast. It is always reliable and can be obtained in most grocery stores. Perhaps more convenient to use is the granular, dry yeast available today in many stores.

In Bible times they used to keep a little dough in an earthen vessel from one baking time to the next. This sour dough was used for yeast in bread making. My mother used this kind of "yeast." Sometimes in the early days we would go to a brewery and for two pennies we would get nearly a two-quart pail full of yeast. This yeast was just the same as the cake yeast today, only it was in liquid form.

From the earliest times a great deal of unleavened bread was used; more, in fact, than leavened bread. The bread that Abraham's wife baked for the mysterious strangers was unleavened bread, for it took her just a short time to make it. In the sacrificial offering no leavened bread was ever used. Leavening was looked upon as a symbol of sin. Indeed, if leavening or yeast of any kind is used in bread, the bread should be thoroughly baked so that the yeast germ is entirely destroyed.

Yeast is sometimes advertised as something to be eaten raw as a stomach remedy but it should never be eaten unless it is first cooked. Yeast is a highly nourishing and wholesome product when it is cooked until the germ is destroyed. In fact, the analysis of yeast is just the same as the analysis of some savory concentrates that are sold for such a high price on the market.

Making Bread Rise

A proper place for bread to rise is of great importance if you would have good bread and have it good every time.

I have sometimes taken an ordinary, clean box, put some shelves in it, and made a door through which I could put my big bread pan. Then I made a place below the lower shelf where I could set a lighted lamp with a little dish of water above it to keep the box an even temperature.

You could put in a large dish of hot water or heat some stones or bricks and wrap in a piece of paper or cloth for the purpose of maintaining an even temperature. There must be considerable space between these stones or bricks and the first shelf upon which your bread is set.

In such a compartment the original sponge can be raised as well as the bread after it is put in pans. In this way you can have good bread every time.

I have also found a common metal grain sprouter very convenient. This may be obtained through farm supply companies. It has a hot water tank over a heating lamp or element which can be regulated to get an even temperature. This is a valuable device to have in order to raise bread and will pay for itself in a short time. You can also use it to make malt, or for sprouting grains and legumes for table use.

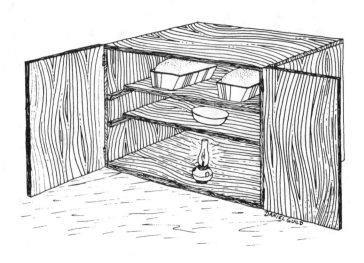

Of course, anyone handy with a saw and hammer could make a wooden box, as previously described, to serve the purpose.

Often people put bread dough on a table somewhere and it gets too cold while it is rising. I never advise that bread be set to rise all night — unless a slow process of rising is made necessary by some special kind of yeast.

Put enough yeast in the bread to make it rise in two or three hours at least. The first time, the dough should rise high enough just before it falls so that when it is touched it will go down. Should it rise so much that it falls of its own accord, it is necessary to reknead it and allow to rise again before it is put into the pans. After it is in the pans, it should rise half its original size before it is put into the oven. If the bread rises too much while in the pan it will be coarse and full of holes. Should it accidentally rise too high, remold it and let it rise again.

Whole wheat flour bread must not be permitted to rise

as light in the pans as white flour bread. Care in this respect will preserve in the bread that sweet, nutty, wheat flavor so characteristic of bread made from the entire grain. It will be lacking if the loaves rise too light in the pans.

Make it a business to have good bread and do not give up until you do. Be determined and say as many others have, "I can make anything that anyone else can."

The Oven

It is important that one have a good oven in order to make good bread. I have found ovens in which the side of the bread nearest the heat would burn; or sometimes it would burn on top, sometimes on the bottom. This problem can be remedied to some extent in most of the ovens by shielding the bread with a sheet of asbestos on the side of the oven that burns.

For whole wheat bread the oven heat should be 450°F, gradually being reduced to 350° or 300°. It is best to use an oven thermometer rather than rely entirely on thermostats. In any case, the oven should be hot enough so the bread will begin to brown in 15 minutes.

Be sure your oven is hot enough. If it is not, your bread will not be good. After the bread is thoroughly heated, reduce the oven temperature, for if the same temperature is maintained after the bread is partly dry, it will burn on the outside. Therefore, the temperature should be gradually reduced from 450 to about 350 degrees and then at last to about 300 or less. Bake your bread thoroughly, allowing at least an hour in the oven.

An Old-Fashioned Clay Oven

Anciently, and even to this day in some lands, people baked bread without an "oven" like ours. Sometimes they baked on the hearth if a fireplace between two hot stones; sometimes in hot ashes or upon the coals. Sometimes they made ovens of clay and straw.

My parents had such an oven, made it in the following fashion. We built a platform about two and a half feet high of two-inch lumber; about five feet wide and six or seven feet long. The boards were heavily covered with clay mixed with cut straw. Then a layer of bricks was laid over the clay so that we had a very smooth surface. Then an arch of wooden slats was built over that. The arch was about two feet high at the center. The back was closed except for a short chimney (which was covered with a small piece of tin to hold the heat after the fire was taken out of the oven). The arch was covered with two or three layers of clay mixed with cut straw. A door was left in front through which the oven was fired and also for putting in and taking out the bread.

A small fire was started in this oven and after the clay was dried a bit and starting to firm up, the fire would be increased in order to burn the clay into brick.

When we wanted to use the oven for bread making, a fire was built in it. When the bread was ready to go into the oven,

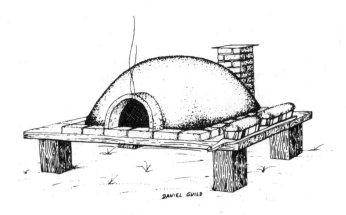

DANIEL GUILD

all the coals and fire were raked out, leaving the hot oven clean and ready for the bread. (We usually let the fire burn long enough to leave the oven "holding" enough heat to bake the bread for an hour to an hour and a half.)

Sometimes we placed the bread right on the brick but we generally put it in pans and baked it as we would in an ordinary oven. This oven baked lovely bread with a beautiful crust. It would be a great blessing if every home had an oven of this kind and more people made their own bread today.

The finest bread may be made in this kind of oven because it bakes just right. The oven should be hot enough so that in 15 minutes the bread will begin to brown. Then allow the heat to gradually diminish as it naturally would in the clay oven after the fire is removed.

Use of Steam in the Oven

It is much easier to get a good crust on bread without burning if there is steam in the oven. This may be accomplished by placing a small pan of water inside. Some commercial bakeries with chain ovens bake under 900 degrees of heat in only 20 to 25 minutes with considerable steam in the oven to keep the bread from burning.

Life-Giving Breads

Whole Wheat Bread

3 cups warm water	1 cake compressed yeast
2 tablespoons honey or natural sugar	7 cups whole wheat flour
	1 tablespoon salt

Dissolve the yeast in a little lukewarm water, add the liquid, and mix all the ingredients to a medium-soft dough. Turn out on a slightly floured board and knead until elastic to the touch; then return to a bowl, cover, and let stand in a warm room to rise until, when tapped sharply, it begins to sink. This takes about two hours.

Work down well, turn over in the bowl, and let rise again one-half its size; then mold into loaves and put into pans. Let rise again until half again its original bulk, then bake in a good oven. Bake at least one hour or longer. These coarse breads must be watched more closely during the rising than those made from white flour, as they get light in much less time.

When taking the baked bread from the oven, sponge it off with a cloth dampened in cold water. Set it in a draft if possible and turn it over to cool quickly so the crust will be brittle and tender. It may be sponged off with a cloth saturated in oil, if desired.

In place of the 3 cups of water, Soy or Nut Milk may be used to improve the bread.

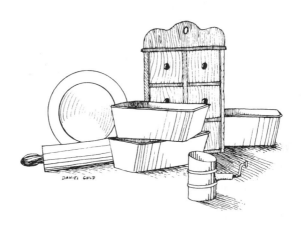

Rye Bread

1 cake compressed yeast	1 cup sifted unbleached
3 cups lukewarm water	white flour
5 cups rye flour	1 tablespoon salt

The white flour should be flour strong in gluten. It should be the same as that used when making washed gluten for nut foods.

Dissolve the yeast in lukewarm water. Add 2 cups of the rye flour, or enough to make a sponge. Beat well. Cover and set aside in a warm place, free from draft, to rise for about two hours.

When light, add the white flour, the rest of the rye flour, or enough to make a soft dough, and the salt. Turn onto a board and knead or pound it for five minutes. Place in a bowl, cover, and let rise until it doubles in bulk. This takes about two hours.

Turn onto board and shape into long loaves. Place in

shallow pans, cover, and let rise again until light about one hour. With a sharp knife cut lightly three strokes diagonally across the top, and place in oven. Bake in a slower oven than for white bread. Caraway seed may be used if desired.

Rye bread can be worked much the same as whole wheat bread. Rye flour does not contain as much gluten and therefore does not rise as light without the addition of wheat flourstrong in gluten.

Whole Wheat Raisin Bread

1 cake compressed yeast	4 tablespoons oil
1 cup lukewarm water	6 cups whole wheat flour
1 teaspoon salt	$3/4$ cup honey or natural sugar
1 cup raw peanut butter	1 cup raisins

Dissolve the yeast in one cup lukewarm water. Add two cups of flour and the sweetening and beat until smooth. Cover and set aside to rise in a warm place, free from any draft, until light about one and one-half hours.

When well-risen, add well-floured raisins, the rest of the flour (or enough to make a moderately soft dough), and the remainder of the ingredients. The raw peanut butter should be first dissolved in a cup of lukewarm water. If the dough is too soft, add a little more flour and next time use less water.

Knead lightly and place in well-greased bowl. Cover and let rise again until double in bulk — about one and one-half hours. Mold into loaves, fill well-greased pans half full, cover, and let rise until light — about one hour. Bake for from one hour to one and a fourth hours.

Steamed Whole Wheat Bread

$3^1/2$ cups whole wheat flour	1 cup Malt Honey or natural
2 cups cornmeal	sugar
3 cups Nut Milk	1 teaspoon salt

Mix the Nut Milk, salt and Malt Honey together; then

mix the corn meal and flour and stir into the liquid. Put into empty cans under five pounds steam pressure and steam for two and one-half or three hours. Then you can put it in the oven and brown it a little for 15 minutes.

Soybean Bread

2 pounds whole wheat flour	1 pint lukewarm water
1 pound soybean mash or	$^{1}/_{2}$ cup malt sugar or honey
$^{1}/_{2}$ pound soy flour	Salt to taste
1 cake compressed yeast	

Dissolve one cake of compressed yeast in a little lukewarm water and add one pint of water. Add the sweetening and salt to taste. Mix this with the flour and soybean mash (with the milk washed out) to make a fairly stiff dough — about the consistency of regular bread dough.

Let it rise to about double its size in a warm place. Then knead it down and lap it over toward the inner side. Turn it over and let it rise again to about half again its size. Then knead it down, mold into loaves and put in pans, letting it rise to about double its size. Bake in a hot oven, about 450 degrees. It should begin to brown about 11 minutes after placing in the oven. Bake the bread thoroughly; this gives it a good flavor and makes it easy to digest.

Diet Soybean Bread

3 pounds whole wheat flour, finely ground	1 cake yeast
	1 pint lukewarm water
1 pound soybean meal (with the milk washed out)	Salt to taste

Mix this together and work it as in regular soybean bread. About 2 or 3 tablespoons of Malt Honey added to the water will add to the flavor and food value. The use of malt extract would make the bread still better because the extract is high in diastase which aids in the digestion of starch.

Diabetics can eat this bread, made into zwieback and

thoroughly dried out until it is a light, golden brown, because the starch has been changed into grape sugar.

Soy Buns or Cinnamon Rolls

4 cups whole wheat flour	1 cup water or Soy Milk
1 cup soybean meal	(see recipe)
½ cup Soy Butter (see recipe)	2 cakes compressed yeast

To the whole wheat flour and the soybean meal, add the Soy Butter. Put in enough yeast so the dough will rise in two or three hours. Mix and knead, turn over and let rise to half gain its size. Now shape into the bun size desired and let rise to about half its bulk again. Bake from 20 to 30 minutes, according to the size of the buns.

Use this mix for cinnamon rolls as you would any dough.

Sesame Cloverleaf Rolls

2 cups hot Soy Milk	6 cups flour, half whole
3 tablespoons oil	wheat and half unbleached
3 tablespoons honey or	white
natural sugar	2 teaspoons salt
1 yeast cake dissolved in	¾ cup sesame seeds
¼ cup lukewarm water	

Add butter, sugar, and salt to Soy Milk. When cooled to lukewarm, add dissolved yeast cake and 3 cups flour. Beat thoroughly, cover, and let rise until light. Cut down and add enough flour to knead (about 2½ cups). Let rise until double in bulk and turn onto slightly floured cloth or board. Knead and shape into tiny balls and roll in sesame seeds. If they don't adhere, moisten ball with a little water.

Place three balls in each section of greased muffin tins. Cover with a cloth and let rise until double in bulk. Bake in hot oven (425°F), 12 to 15 minutes. Brush lightly with oil.

Old-Fashioned Beaten Biscuits

2 cups whole wheat flour

²/₃ cup Soy Milk (see recipe)

¹/₂ cup Soy Butter (see recipe)

Salt

2 tablespoons honey

Put flour into a bowl, add the Soy Milk, then the Soy Butter and salt. Mix into a stiff dough as you would in making ordinary bread. Beat with a rolling pin or any heavy stick. This beating is done to make the biscuit tender and mellow.

Make into sticks or roll about one-half inch thick and cut in sizes to suit your taste. This can be rolled still thinner and made into a cracker if you like. Prick with a fork to keep it from blistering. Bake in a very hot oven to a light brown.

Let me tell you a little more about how I make beaten

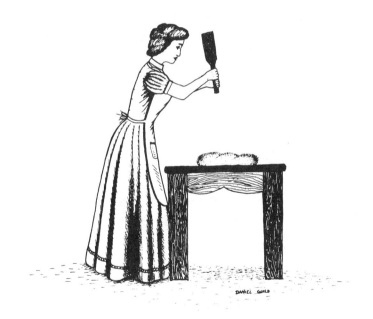

biscuits. I make a table top of cement — 6 inches thick, 18 inches wide, and 2 feet long; or you could make it of heavy planks. Then, with a piece of two-by-four about three feet long, I beat the dough, folding it over and over; repeating the folding and beating. I beat it until it is flattened out, then fold it over and beat some more, repeating the process at least 20 times or more. This would depend on the weight of the beater and the vigor put into the beating!

After the dough has been well-beaten (about 10 or 15 minutes), I make it into little biscuits or cut it thin into little crackers or sticks.

When it is baked long enough to be thoroughly dextrinized it will be mellow enough to melt in your mouth. It makes one of the finest, most easily digested breads that can be made — without any shortening, baking powder, soda, or yeast. (A little shortening may be used, such as Soy Butter as given in this book — if you wish to use shortening.)

These are old-fashioned beaten biscuits! This method would also produce a very fine pie crust. (Always use whole wheat flour to make old-fashioned beaten biscuits.)

Corn Bread

2 cups yellow corn meal
1 cup finely grated carrots
3 tablespoons oil
1 teaspoon salt
2 tablespoons natural sugar
  or honey
1 1/2 cups boiling water

Mix corn meal, sweetening, salt, and oil. Pour in boiling water. Add carrots and mix well. Pour into oiled pan and bake one hour at 450°F, then half an hour at 400°F. (To predextrinize the corn meal, see recipe for Olden Days Corn-Soy Muffins.)

Corn Pone

1/3 pound corn meal
1/3 pound whole wheat flour
1/3 pound oatmeal flour
1 1/2 cups Soy Milk or water
2 tablespoons Malt Honey or
  natural sugar

Mix all together. Have batter cold; pans and oven hot. Bake 30 minutes, more or less, depending on the heat of the oven.

Special Corn Pone

1/2 cup honey	3 cups corn meal
1/2 teaspoon salt	2 tablespoons oil
1 cup unbleached flour	1 cup Soy Milk
1 tablespoon soy flour	

Mix, beat well, and drop the batter from spoon in flat cakes and bake in hot oven about 25 minutes.

Corn Dodgers

2 cups corn meal	1/4 cup honey
1 1/2 tablespoons oil	1 cup boiling water
1 teaspoon salt	3/4 cup Soy Milk

Add oil to mixed, dry ingredients. Add boiling water all at once. Add Soy Milk and stir until smooth. Add just enough milk to make batter drop from spoon but not run. Drop mixture from large spoon onto oiled baking pan and bake in hot oven.

Zwieback

Bread baked in the ordinary way is never entirely dextrinized, or the starch turned into grape sugar.

Zwieback (or twice-baked bread) is, and is thus very wholesome and easy to digest.

To make zwieback, slice the bread about three-fourths of an inch thick and let it dry out in the sun, or slow oven, until it is entirely dry. Increase the temperature of the oven and make the bread a golden brown. It must be carefully watched as it burns easily.

I have kept zwieback in fine shape for an entire year in a common barrel lined with heavy brown paper. During this time there was a long period of wet weather and it seemed as if the zwieback had gathered a little moisture but there was not a trace of mold. I put it outdoors on paper in the sun and let it dry out thoroughly. After it had been heated in the oven, it was just as good as when freshly made.

Zwieback should be an important part of our diet. It can save a great deal of time and expense. Use for breakfast or lunch. For an excellent lunch, serve it with fruits or fruit juices, Soy Milk or Malted Nut Cream. Use it any way you like but make it a practice to have a large supply of zwieback on hand.

Health Muffins or Crackers

Muffins for those suffering with Bright's disease, diabetes, liver or kidney troubles may be made in the following way.

Put whole wheat flour in a pan on the stove. Stir frequently with a wooden paddle until it is very slightly golden brown — at a stage we call dextrinized.

Mix 2 cups of the flour, 1 cup of soy flour, 1 cup of boiled spinach or 1 cup of powdered spinach. Add peanut milk made from raw peanut butter (mix raw peanut butter into a cream with water to the consistency of thin cream or cows milk).

Beat the batter just thick enough so it will drop from a spoon, and salt to taste.

If you wish to make crackers, more flour should be added. Roll it out to any thickness you want and cut it to any size you desire.

This makes a wonderful product, either as a cracker or a muffin.

Carrots may be used in place of spinach. You may also add 2 tablespoons of Malt Honey or natural sugar.

Unleavened Muffins

To make unleavened bread with any kind of meal, the whole thing in a nutshell is this:

Have your water and Nut Milk as cold as possible, salted

to taste. Add a little Soy Butter and a little honey, if desired. Have your muffin pans sizzling hot and your batter just stiff enough so that it will drop from the spoon. Place in the oven and bake. This will make a very palatable bread.

Cornmeal Muffins

1 cup corn meal	2 tablespoons oil
1 cup whole wheat flour	1 teaspoon salt
1 cup Soy Milk (see recipe)	

Mix the milk, oil, and salt in a bowl. Beat the flour into this mixture. The ingredients should be cold as described above and your muffin pans sizzling hot. Bake in very hot oven.

Oatmeal or Soybean Muffins

1 cup corn meal	1½ cups Soy Milk
1 cup whole wheat flour	(see recipe)
1 cup oatmeal or	3 tablespoons oil
soybean meal	1 teaspoon salt

Follow directions for making Cornmeal Muffins.

Potato or Carrot Muffins

2 cups whole wheat flour	1 cup Soy Milk (see recipe)
1 cup mashed Irish potatoes,	3 tablespoons oil
sweet potatoes, or	Salt to taste
mashed carrots	

Follow directions for making Cornmeal Muffins. In place of oil in the three recipes above, Soy Butter may be used for a better product because the oil is emulsified and more easily digested.

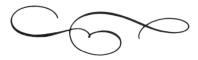

Olden Days Corn-Soy Muffins

¹/₂ pound soybean mash (with milk washed out)	¹/₂ pound dextrinized corn meal (see below)
¹/₂ cup Soy Milk or water	

To dextrinize the corn meal place it in the oven in a large baking pan. Stir frequently with a pancake turner or a wooden paddle until it is a golden brown. Do not have the oven so hot as to burn the meal. This procedure turns the corn starch into dextrose and makes it palatable and easy of digestion.

Mix the soybean mash and the dextrinized corn meal with the Soy Milk. Salt to taste. Pour the mix into hot, cast-iron muffin pans and bake for 20 minutes in a hot oven.

This makes a very wholesome muffin — one that diabetics can eat.

This mixture made thinner with more milk may be poured out in dots on a pan as drop cookies and baked in a very hot oven.

Crisp Whole Wheat Crackers

1 pound whole wheat flour	¹/₂ pint water
5 ounces raw peanut butter	Salt

Dissolve the peanut butter in the water stir in the flour and salt to taste. Make the dough stiff enough to be rolled. This makes a lovely cracker.

It can be improved by adding to your peanut milk about two big tablespoons of Malt Honey or other natural sweetener. This is a complete food and very palatable.

These crackers may also be made from raised dough. Make the dough as for bread. Take a scant 1 pint of water, a 1 pound of Malt Honey or other sweetener, and about 4 ounces of raw peanut butter. Make the peanut butter into a milk and set the sponge as for bread. Use for this amount about 1 cake of compressed yeast. When the mix has risen, as for bread, knead it and work it into thin rolls. Prick them with a fork so they will not blister. Cut into strips and bake until brown. This makes a very delicious cracker.

Raised Oatmeal Crackers

6 pounds finely ground oatmeal flour	1 1/2 pounds Malt Honey, malt sugar, or other natural sugar
3 pounds unbleached pastry flour	2 ounces compressed yeast
2 cups oil	2 quarts water
1 ounce salt	

Mix the oil with the flour, rubbing well, then add water. The sweetening should be dissolved in the water before mixing with flour. Roll very thin, less than one-fourth inch, and bake in hot oven until light brown.

Soy-Oat Crackers

2 cups hot Soy Milk or Nut Milk (enough to make a thick batter)	4 cups hot ground oatmeal

After mixing ingredients, allow to stand 20 to 30 minutes. Roll out the dough to about one-eighth inch thickness (using whole wheat flour on board). Cut into desired wafer size. Place on oiled cookie sheet and bake 15 minutes in moderate oven. Should be slightly brown, dry, and hard. Will keep several weeks in closed container.

Rye Crisps

A good crisp, rye cracker can be made very easily at home. Use whole rye flour with enough water to make a dough stiff enough to be rolled. Add a little salt and then bake 15 or 20 minutes in a hot oven. These crackers are very wholesome but cannot or should not be swallowed without thorough mastication.

Whole Wheat Sticks

4 cups whole wheat flour	1 tablespoon salt
2/3 cup natural sugar or honey	1 1/4 cups chopped nuts
2/3 cup oil	1 cup cold water

Combine all ingredients, using only enough water to make a stiff dough — one cup should be about right. Knead until dough is uniform, like bread dough. Then roll on a large cookie sheet to about half-inch thickness and cut into sticks. Bake in moderate oven until done and well-browned.

Coconut-Wheat Sticks

2 cups whole wheat flour	4 tablespoons natural sugar
1/3 cup chopped nuts	or honey
1/3 cup coconut	5 tablespoons oil
1/2 teaspoon salt	1/2 cup water

Mix dry ingredients. Add oil and mix. Add nuts and coconut and mix. Gradually add water until dough is stiff. Knead. Press out with hands to half-inch thickness on cookie sheet. Cut into sticks. Bake 30 minutes in moderate oven. Roll or turn once or twice during baking, if needed.

Natural Breakfast Foods

Browned and Steamed Rice

1 cup natural brown rice   ½ teaspoon salt
3½ cups water

Put rice in a covered frying pan and stir over fire until light brown in color. Add boiling water and boil until dry and tender. Let stand a few minutes before serving. Rice improves if your cooking pan, covered, stands in another pan of boiling water for 10 to 15 minutes.

Rice prepared in this way has enhanced flavor and digestibility and can be used as boiled rice in many recipes.

Chinese Boiled Rice

Wash thoroughly 1 cup of natural, brown rice and place in a heavy, deep kettle with a tight-fitting lid. Add water to cover rice about an inch and a half. Bring to a boil. Turn down the heat and simmer for 20 minutes. Do not stir or open lid. Rice should be dry and fluffy. It will remain hot in the kettle for several hours.

Fluffy Soft Rice

1 cup natural brown rice   5 cups boiling water
1 1/2 teaspoons salt

Add washed rice to boiling, salted water and boil slowly for 10 to 15 minutes. Cover and place in a hot oven for 30 minutes.

Slow-Cooked Breakfast Rice

1 cup natural brown rice   Salt to taste
4 cups water

After washing the rice, place it in the boiling, salted water, stirring until it rolls up in a rapid boil. Let it continue boiling in this way until it swells, then set onto the lower part of a double boiler and cook more slowly. Do not stir after it begins to swell. It will require one hour or more to thoroughly cook brown rice. The kernels should be very tender.

Soy Baked Rice

1/2 to 3/4 cup natural   2 cups Soy Milk
    brown rice   1/2 teaspoon salt

Wash and drain the rice. Heat the Soy Milk, pour into a baking dish, and add the rice. Cover and bake in a slow oven two to three hours without stirring, or until the milk is thickened and creamy with rice. If the milk boils out under the cover, the oven is too hot.

This makes a very delicious dish, for breakfast or any meal, and does not require any additions. However, if a dressing is desired, Milk Sweetening, the recipe for which is given in this book, may be diluted with a little water or Soy Milk and poured over the rice. Fig Marmalade (see Fig Marmalade Pie) may be diluted and served with it.

An excellent rice pudding can be made by adding 1/2 cup Malt Honey or honey and 1 cup of raisins just before placing the rice in the oven to bake.

Breakfast Wheat

1 cup whole grain wheat	A few grains of salt
3 cups water	

Place in a double boiler and cook until the kernels burst. Raisins, stoned dates, or chopped figs may be stirred into the wheat just before serving. These give natural sweetness and are far better for the system than adding sugar to cereals.

The wheat can also be cooked in a steam pressure cooker until the kernels are done, about one hour, or in a crock in the oven. Set the crock in a pan of water to keep the wheat from burning. This requires about four hours.

Cornmeal Mush

1 cup corn meal	$3/4$ cup cold water
$2^{1}/_{2}$ cups boiling water	1 teaspoon salt

Blend the corn meal with the cold water. Blend mix into

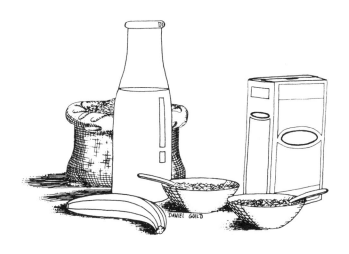

the boiling water and stir until it boils. Boil rapidly until it begins to thicken. Place it in double boiler and cook until thoroughly done.

The Original Granola

Mix with whole wheat flour and enough water to make a stiff dough. Roll it out about a quarter or half an inch thick. Put it in the oven and bake until it is partly dextrinized, nearly a golden brown. Take a mallet and break it up, then put it through a grinder. After grinding, put it in a baking pan and reheat to dextrinize it slightly more.

Kloss' Granola

2 cups whole wheat flour	1 cup soybean mash (or 1 cup
Soy Milk	soy flour)

Prepare this in the same way as The Original Granola, using enough Soy Milk to make a stiff dough.

Granola Supreme

First, mix these ingredients:

1¹/₂ cup whole wheat flour	¹/₂ cup corn meal
1¹/₂ cups rolled oats	¹/₂ cup fresh wheat germ
¹/₂ cup soy flour	¹/₂ cup coconut meal or
¹/₂ cup rye flour	grated coconut
¹/₄ cup millet meal	¹/₂ cup sesame seed

Then mix in a blender these ingredients:

¹/₄ to ¹/₃ cup water	¹/₂ cup oil
¹/₄ cup pecans	¹/₂ cup honey
¹/₄ cup almonds	1 teaspoon salt

Combine the two mixtures and mix thoroughly. Bake one hour in a slow oven, stirring every 10 to 15 minutes to keep separated into small bits.

Old-Fashioned Granola

1 cup whole wheat flour	1 cup cottonseed meal
1 cup corn meal	

Mix and prepare in the same way as The Original Granola.

The mix for granola recipes can be raised with yeast and baked into loaves of bread. When a day or two old, the loaves can be broken up while the bread is still a little moist and run through a mill, then put in a baking pan and reheated.

Original Dixie Kernel

1 cup corn meal	1 cup oatmeal
1 cup whole wheat flour	1 cup finely ground bran
1 teaspoonful salt	

Mix these ingredients and add enough water to make a stiff dough. Roll out to about one-half inch thickness. Bake in a moderate oven until slightly browned. When it is a day old, grind up while still a little moist.

Add 1 cup of water to 1 cup of Malt Honey, mixing thoroughly. Sprinkle this over the ground cereal product. Do not let the mixture get too moist. Now spread it out to partly dry and then place in an oven to dextrinize, making it a slight golden brown.

This is a very delicate and tasty breakfast food.

Old-Fashioned Dixie Kernel

Take various kinds of bread and broken crackers — such as bran, whole wheat, oatmeal — and grind them together.

Take equal parts of Malt Honey or honey and water, stirring well together, and sprinkle over the ground material, mixing it up thoroughly to slightly moisten it. Place in the oven, stir frequently to prevent burning, and slightly dextrinize to a golden brown.

This makes a very delightful breakfast food.

Kloss' Soy-Corn Pancakes

1 cup corn meal	1 cup soybean mash
1 cup Soy Milk (see recipe)	½ cup Malt Sugar or honey
½ cup Soy Butter (see recipe)	Salt to taste

To the corn meal and soybean mash add the Soy Milk and beat up as ordinary pancake batter. Add the sweetener, salt, and beat in the Soy Butter.

If the batter is used when very cold, the pancakes can be made nicely without yeast or baking powder. If the pancakes are for breakfast, it is well to soak the corn meal in the Soy Milk the night before.

Some like the pancakes made with yeast. Dissolve one cake of yeast in the Soy Milk and proceed as above, letting it rise about an hour before baking.

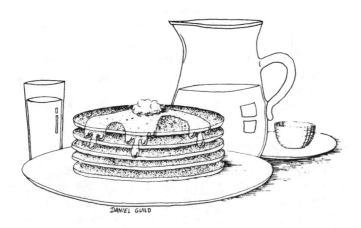

DANIEL GUILD

Kloss' Eggless French Toast

Slice soy bread about one-half inch thick and let dry in the sun or a moderately warm oven. When thoroughly dry, increase the heat in the oven enough to brown it a golden color clear through. This browning turns the starch into dextrose or grape sugar, making it almost like the juice in ripe fruit.

Now immerse the toast in Soy Milk, being careful not to leave it too long. Lift out with a pancake turner, and spread a thin coating of Substitute for Egg Yolks (see recipe) on each slice. Have your frying pan hot with a little oil on it, place the toast in with the side down that has the "egg yolk" spread on it. Now, put spread on the top side, leaving until the underside is browned, then turn it over until the top side is browned.

Serve wih diluted Malt Honey, honey, or maple syrup. French toast with a cup of hot Soy Milk is nice for a light supper.

This toast makes a wholesome and easily digested dish, containing all the necessary food elements.

Soups...Total Nutrition

No wonder that in situations of severe food scarcity the most common forms of prepared foods are breads or cereals and soups or stews. All the nutrients can be conserved and utilized in these forms of food preparation.

In soups, one eats with pleasure the savory nutrients that otherwise might be discarded in the cooking of vegetables, legumes, or fruits.

Here are many soup suggestions for pleasant, total nutrition — food scarcity or not.

Bean Soup

1½ cups beans, any kind
1 large tomato, peeled and diced (or use tomato sauce or canned tomatoes)
1 teaspoon Savory Seasoning (see recipe)
1 tablespoon salt

3 small onions, finely chopped
1 clove garlic, finely chopped (or garlic powder)
½ teaspoon paprika
4 cups water, more or less

Cook beans, and when nearly done add salt and tomato. In a skillet, sauté onions and garlic in a little oil and add paprika and Savory Seasoning. Combine all ingredients, cover, and simmer for one hour, stirring occasionally. Add additional water, if needed, and season to taste. A good hearty soup.

Hot or Cold Borsch

2 cups shredded beets
1 cup chopped carrots
1 cup chopped onions
1 cup coarsely chopped
  cabbage

1 tablespoon oil
1 tablespoon lemon juice
Soy Butter
Savory Vegetable Extract
  (see recipe)

Cook covered the beets, carrots, and chopped onions in 5 cups boiling salted water. This takes about 20 minutes.

Add Savory Seasoning to taste, the chopped cabbage, and oil. Cook uncovered for 15 minutes.

Stir in lemon juice and add any other seasonings desired. Serve hot or cold topped with a spoonful of Soy Butter or sour cream.

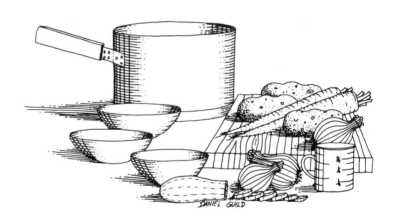

DANIEL GUILD

Cream of Corn Soup

2 cups fresh or canned corn   6 cups rich Soy Milk
Salt to taste   (see recipe)

Heat the milk, put the corn through a sieve, add to hot milk, salt to taste, and serve.

Eggplant Soup

3 cups diced eggplant   2 cups Soy Milk (see recipe)
3 cups water

Cook the eggplant in the water until tender, then add the Soy Milk, salt to taste, and add one tablespoon Soy Butter while very hot, just before serving.

Golden Soup

2 cups thinly sliced carrots   5 cups cold water
2 cups thinly sliced raw   1 cup Soy Milk
   potato   Salt
2 stalks of celery (cut in   1 tablespoon oil
   small pieces)   1 large sprig parsley
1 small sliced onion

Put carrots, onion, parsley, and oil into a saucepan. Add half a cup of water. Cover and cook slowly until dry, stirring now and then to prevent burning. Add water, potato, celery, salt, and boil rapidly. Put through a sieve. Add the hot milk, and strain again. Salt to taste.

Cream of Lentil Soup

4 cups water   2 cups rich Soy Milk
3 cups cooked lentils   Parsley
  (sprouted preferable)

Put the lentils through a sieve, add the Soy Milk and 1 quart of water; salt to taste. Season with onion and a little savory Vegetable Extract. Just before serving, add finely cut parsley and 2 tablespoons Soy Butter.

Rich Lentil Soup

2 cups cooked lentils
1/4 cup chopped cooked
   carrots
1/4 cup chopped green onions

1 cup tomato juice
2 cups lentil juice
1/2 cup finely cut parsley

Mix all the ingredients, heat to the boiling point, add 1 tablespoon Soy Butter, salt to taste, and serve.

Lentil-Herb Soup

PART I
1 cup dry lentils
5 cups water
1/8 teaspoon oregano
1/8 teaspoon thyme
1 tablespoon salt

PART II
1 onion or 3 green onions,
   chopped and sautéed
1 carrot, grated
1/4 cup chopped parsley
1/4 cup oil

Cook slowly in separate covered pans for 15 minutes. Combine the two parts.

Add 1 or 2 chopped tomatoes or a small can of whole tomatoes. Boil all ingredients together for 45 minutes or until lentils are tender.

Bean-Rich Minestrone

1/2 cup pinto beans
1/2 cup garbanzos
1/2 cup northern white beans
1/2 cup lima beans
1/2 cup pink beans
1/2 cup red beans
1/2 cup olive oil
1 large chopped onion

1 clove chopped garlic
2 cups celery and leaves,
   chopped
1 No. 2 1/2 can whole tomatoes
   cut in pieces
1/4 cup chopped parsley
2 cups shredded cabbage
6 zucchini squash, thinly sliced

Soak all the beans overnight in 10 cups of water. (Add more as needed to keep beans covered.) Cook beans two or three hours or until done.

Sauté onion, garlic, and parsley in olive oil. Add sautéed

vegetables, cut up tomatoes, and parsley to the cooked beans. Simmer covered for 45 minutes.

Add cabbage, squash, and enough water to yield 7½ quarts of soup. Cook until cabbage and squash are done.

Serve hot or refrigerate or freeze so that you may have a supply on hand.

Cream of Lettuce and Potato Soup

1 cup shredded lettuce	1 tablespoon chopped onion
2 cups sliced raw potato	1½ teaspoons salt
4 cups cold water	1 cup Soy Milk

Put the potato, onion, and salt in the water and bring to a boil. When the potato is about half done, add the lettuce and boil rapidly until the vegetables are well-cooked. Press through a colander. Add the hot Soy Milk and mix. Salt to taste, put through a sieve and serve.

Potato-Onion Soup

6 medium-sized potatoes (with peeling), sliced fine	5 tablespoons chopped parsley
3 large onions, cut fine	2 quarts water

Combine ingredients and simmer for an hour. Add 1 heaping tablespoon each of soybean flour and oat flour, mixed thoroughly with a little cold water. Boil five minutes.

Soy Butter can be used in place of the soybean and oat flours, adding 1 heaping tablespoon to the soup just before serving. Use salt moderately.

Cream of Spinach Soup

1 cup cooked spinach pulp	1 cup mashed potatoes
2 cups rich Soy Milk	2 cups potato water

Mix the spinach pulp and Soy Milk, add the mashed potatoes (made as described in this book), and potato water, salt to taste, bring to a boil, add 1 tablespoon Soy Butter.

Old-Fashioned Stew

1 cup chopped onions	½ teaspoon salt
2 tablespoons oil	⅛ teaspoon garlic powder
1 can vegetable or nut roast (see recipes)	2 carrots, cut in strips
	½ cup sliced celery
1½ cups hot water	2 cups cubed potatoes
Savory Seasoning to taste (see recipes)	½ cup canned tomato pieces
	2 sprigs parsley, chopped

Put oil in large, heavy saucepan. Add onions and cook at medium heat until tender. Add water and seasonings and bring to a boil. Add carrots and celery and cook 10 minutes. Add potatoes and nut roast (diced) and cook 10 minutes longer. Stir in tomatoes and parsley and simmer until well blended.

Tomato Soup

1 quart water	1 tablespoon oil
1 tablespoon quick oats	Salt to taste
4 cups tomato pieces	

Cook the oats in boiling water 10 minutes. Put the tomatoes through flour sieve; add to water and oil. Boil five minutes. Salt and add a little Soy Mayonnaise before serving.

Rich Tomato Soup

3 cups rich tomato juice	3 heaping tablespoons
3 cups cold water	soy flour

Mix the tomato juice and water and bring to a boil. Make a thin paste of the soy flour mixed with cold water. Stir this into the hot tomato juice and let simmer five minutes. A heaping tablespoon of Soy Butter may be added. (Dilute the butter in a little cold water and put through a fine sieve before adding to the soup.) Let the soup get real hot, add a pinch of salt, and serve.

All nut milks may be used in place of Soy Milk. Flavor with a little soy sauce if desired, to taste.

Cream of Tomato Soup

1 quart Soy Milk   Salt to taste
2 cups tomato juice

Boil milk for two or three minutes. Let it cool a little, add the tomato juice and a little Soy Mayonnaise (see recipe) and salt. Serve hot.

Do not boil the soup after the tomatoes are added. It can be reheated but do not boil.

More tomato juice may be added if a stronger tomato flavor is desired.

Oatmeal water made with four parts of water to one part of oatmeal soaked overnight and then strained is an excellent addition to any soup stock. It increases the vitamins and makes the soup creamy.

Rich Cream of Tomato Soup

6 cups very rich Soy Milk   6 heaping tablespoons soy
   (see recipe)   flour (make into a thin
6 cups rich tomato juice   paste with cold water)

Heat the tomato juice; add the soy flour paste, stirring constantly. Do not let it boil; just simmer. In five minutes, stir the thickened tomato juice into the hot milk, heat a few minutes, add a pinch of salt, and serve.

You may also use a milk made from any nuts in place of Soy Milk. Milk made from raw peanut butter is excellent;

Pioneer Vegetable Soup

Use 1 cup each of carrots, cabbage, celery; ½ cup onions and potatoes (do not peel the potatoes but scrub with a wire brush so the eyes will remain in the potatoes — they are the life-giving part). Add two quarts or so of water.

After all this has come to a boil, add 1 cup of brown rice and simmer slowly one to two hours or more. Salt to taste.

When soup is done take off the heat and add 1 quart Soy Milk — more or less to suit the taste.

(Be sure to use the green leaves of the celery and cabbage. The green leaves of cauliflower are better still — and these are usually thrown away.)

If the soup is to be fed to invalids, or those who have ulcers, cancer of the stomach, or to small children, let it simmer slowly at least two and a half or three hours. Then mash the vegetables with a wire potato masher and let boil a few minutes longer. Strain through a fine wire strainer. When all this is done, add the Soy Milk. This is a wonderful alkaline dish and highly nourishing. Tomato juice may be added instead of the Soy Milk if you like.

The cold soup is a very nourishing drink and very high in vitamins and other life-giving properties — generally far superior to sauerkraut juice or tomato juice.

You can add different kinds of green vegetables to suit your own taste; or you may use more of one kind and less of others.

Robust Vegetable Soup

2 large carrots (do not peel)	Medium bunch of celery
4 turnips	(using leaves)
4 onions	1 cup lima beans
Parsley (use generously)	1 cup green peas (or 1 cup
Green leaves of cabbage,	purée of dry split peas
chopped	and lima beans)

If you do not like onion, use soy sauce for flavoring, to suit your taste.

Cut the vegetables in small pieces and let them simmer until cooked soft. Do not boil hard. Add a little salt when finished.

To repeat, soups can be made from any combination of vegetables one likes: celery, carrots, potatoes, parsley, onions, okra are very good. You may add beans — such as navy, lima, marrow-beans, green split peas — soaked overnight, cooked very slowly until thoroughly done, then put through a fine sieve or colander. (If this sifted pulp is too thick, thin with soy or nut milk.)

Flavor with onion, garlic, or parsley, cut very fine and added to the sifted pulp. Heat about 10 minutes before serving. Use salt moderately. Never use black or white pepper. Cayenne (red pepper), is good.

Year-Round Fruit Soup

(My parents used a great deal of fruit soup when I was a child.)

2 cups raisins	1 cup unsweetened
2 cups prunes	grape juice
2 lemons	4 quarts cold water

Use Malt Sugar or honey to sweeten to taste.

Add raisins and prunes to the water and let them simmer until done. (It is good to first soak them overnight in the water; then they need very little cooking.) Add the grape juice and lemon, sliced very thin, and the sweetening to taste. This can be served hot or cold as you desire.

Important — Do not serve this soup with a vegetable meal. Use it with whole wheat zwieback, whole wheat crackers — or any of the whole grain products — soy muffins, nut products, or nuts. Used in this way it makes a fine luncheon or fruit meal.

Tropical Fruit Soup

2 tablespoons tapioca	½ cup orange sections
1½ cups water	cut in half
1 tablespoon honey or	1½ cups sliced fresh or
natural sugar	canned peaches
Dash of salt	2-3 medium-sized bananas,
1 6-ounce can concentrated	diced
orange juice	

Combine tapioca and water and let stand for 15 minutes. Cook and stir this mixture over medium heat until it comes to a boil.

Remove from heat and mix in the sweetening, salt, and orange juice (undiluted). Cool, stirring after 15 minutes, then cover and chill.

Before serving, fold in orange sections, peaches, and bananas.

Fresh Vegetable Minestrone

1 beet (beet cubed, leaves chopped)
1 cup diced carrots
1 cup young green beans
1 cup diced turnips
1 small cabbage (soaked 10 minutes in salt water, chop evenly)
1/2 cup sliced green squash
1/2 cup chopped onions or leeks
1 cup diced celery

1/2 cup chopped tender spinach leaves
1/2 cup fresh parsley
1 clove garlic
1 1/2 cups tomato pieces
1 tablespoon salt
1 teaspoon chopped basil
4 or 5 bay leaves (remove before serving)
Savory Vegetable Extract to taste
2 quarts water

2 cans Heinz vegetarian beans

Combine all ingredients in a large kettle and bring to a boil. Cover and cook slowly for an hour and a half.

If you use canned or frozen vegetables, add them in last half of cooking time.

In the last 15 minutes of cooking time, add 2 cans of Heinz vegetarian beans.

Grandmother Kloss' Split Pea Soup

2 cups dry green split peas
1 stalk celery, chopped
1 large carrot, chopped
2 quarts water

1 small onion, chopped
1/4 teaspoon thyme
1 bay leaf
Salt to taste

Combine all ingredients and boil for 20 minutes. Reduce the heat and simmer an hour or more until the peas are done. Strain through colander and serve.

Creamy Split Pea Soup

Use green or yellow split peas. Cook and press through a sieve. To the pea purée add rich Soy Milk until you have the desired consistency. Some gluten, diced very small, will add greatly to this soup. Season with onions, garlic, parsley, or soy sauce. Vegetable Extract may also be used (see recipe).

Rich Potato Soup

3 cups mashed potatoes	2 cups rich Soy Milk
2 tablespoons chopped onions	1 quart water
	Parsley or watercress

Make the mashed potatoes by the recipe in the book. Mix ingredients together, bring to a boil, add 1 tablespoon Soy Butter and serve.

Salads and Dressings

Salads are refreshing and life-giving with any combination of vegetables — if they are fresh and crisp.

Do not combine fruits and vegetables in the same salad; it is not a healthful combination. Serve vegetable salads with vegetable meals; or, make a nourishing vegetable salad and serve with nuts or some good meat substitute for luncheon. At another time have a fruit salad with nuts or some good meat substitute for luncheon or with a fruit meal.

Do not use commercial mayonnaise or any other dressing that has vinegar, mustard, black or white pepper, or refined sugar in it. Make your own healthful mayonnaise if you wish to use mayonnaise (see recipes).

Here are some other dressings that are healthful and refreshing.

Golden Salad Dressing

1 cup carrot juice	1 cup soy oil
1/2 cup soy powder	1 teaspoon salt
1/2 cup crushed pineapple	2 tablespoons lemon juice

Blend the carrot juice, soy powder, and pineapple. Mixing with an eggbeater, pour in the oil in a very fine stream. When thickened, add the salt and lemon juice and blend.

Green Pepper Salad Dressing

1 large green pepper
6 small green onions or
    1/2 Spanish onion
Lemon juice, if desired

4 tablespoons Soy Mayonnaise
    (see recipe)
3 tablespoons Healthful
    Ketchup (see recipe)

Chop pepper and onions very fine, mix all ingredients, and refrigerate for two hours.

Lemon-Honey Dressing

1 teaspoon honey
1/4 cup oil

2 tablespoons lemon juice

Mix thoroughly and use with any kind of salad greens.

Lemon-Honey French Dressing

1/2 cup oil
1/4 cup lemon juice
2 tablespoons honey

1/2 teaspoon each celery salt,
    onion salt, paprika
1/2 cup tomato sauce

Mix thoroughly before serving.

Soy Salad Dressing

1/2 cup rich Soy Milk
1 cup soy oil
1/4 cup lemon juice

1 tablespoon sesame seed
    meal
1 tablespoon honey

Add oil to Soy Milk, gradually while mixing. Add sesame seed meal and beat until thickened. Add lemon juice and honey. Season to taste (onion, celery, garlic).

Sweet-and-Sour Dressing

1/2 cup Soy Mayonnaise
2 tablespoons lemon juice

2 to 3 teaspoons honey
1/2 cup Soy Cream or Soy Milk

Mix thoroughly and serve with shredded lettuce and sliced onions — or any favorite salad mix.

Special Diet Dressing

3 tablespoons lemon juice	3 teaspoons honey
7 tablespoons tomato juice	1 teaspoon salt
1/2 cup water	2 tablespoons soy flour

Cook in double boiler until thick. Cook and place in a tightly closed jar and keep refrigerated until you wish to serve it.

Avocado-Stuffed Celery

1 ripe avocado, mashed	3 ounces Soy Cheese
1/4 cup chopped onions	1 teaspoon seasoned salt

Combine and use to fill 12 to 16 2-inch pieces of celery. Top with slices of green olive.

Carrousel Bean Salad

Equal parts	1/2 chopped bell pepper
(about 2 cups each):	3-4 chopped green onions
green beans,	1/2 cup honey or natural sugar
kidney beans,	1/3 cup oil
wax beans,	1/3 cup lemon juice
garbanzos	Salt and garlic to taste

Combine all ingredients. (If canned beans are used, drain first.) Cover and place in refrigerator several hours before serving.

Garden Salad

1 cup diced cooked carrots	3 cups tomato pieces
1 diced cooked cauliflower	1 chopped cucumber
1 cup cooked peas	1 cup chopped lettuce
1 cup chopped cooked celery	

Serve with dressing and sprinkle with chopped nuts. The same vegetables may be used raw for even better nutrition.

Lettuce Salad Rolls

1 cup Soy Cottage Cheese	½ cup chopped nuts
½ cup chopped dates	1 teaspoon grated orange peel

Combine and spread onto small pieces of lettuce leaf. Roll like a jelly roll and fasten with toothpicks.

Kloss Potato Salad

Potato	Celery
Onion (green preferred)	Cucumbers
Parsley	Ripe olives

Prepare the potatoes by boiling with the skins on. Dry out when done so they are light and mealy. Cool the potatoes and skin them, making your salad for use immediately if you wish the best flavor.

Chop the onions, celery, and ripe olives quite fine. Mince

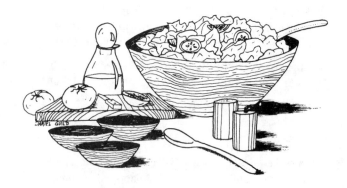

the parsley and mix with diced cucumbers and potatoes. Leave the skin on the cucumber if it is a nice thin skin. Salt moderately, add finely chopped nuts and a pinch of cayenne.

Mix with Soy Mayonnaise and garnish with radishes and parsley.

Never use stale potatoes in making potato salad; it is much better to have them freshly cooked.

High Protein Salad

1 cup vegetarian roast of your choice (see recipe)
1 cup cooked green peas
1 cup diced celery
1 tablespoon lemon juice
1 tablespoon grated onion
Salt to taste
Soy Mayonnaise (see recipe)

Cut roast into small cubes and brown lightly in a little oil. Cool and combine with peas, celery, grated onion, lemon juice, salt, and Soy Mayonnaise. Serve on lettuce leaf. Garnish with tomatoes and sprigs of parsley, if desired.

Red, White, and Green Salad

1 No. 2 can red kidney beans
1 small green pepper, chopped
1 small onion, chopped fine
1 to 2 tablespoons Soy Mayonnaise (see recipe)
1/4 cup lemon juice

Mix beans, pepper, and onion. Blend Soy Mayonnaise and lemon juice and pour over the other ingredients. Toss well and serve on a bed of lettuce.

Soybean Salad

1 1/2 cups cooked soybeans
1/2 cup diced celery
1/4 cup dressing (Lemon-Honey French Dressing is good)
1/2 cup diced Soy Cheese (see recipe)
1/2 cup diced carrots
1 teaspoon finely minced onion

Mix with salad dressing. Chill and serve on lettuce.

Tomato Aspic Salad

6 cups fresh or canned tomatoes	2 teaspoons salt
8 bay leaves	2 teaspoons celery salt
3 small onions	2 packages vegetable gelatin (agar-agar)

Cook tomatoes, onions, and seasoning until reduced one-half. Add vegetable gelatin and boil. Rub through a sieve to remove seeds. Pour into six molds moistened with cold water. Chill and unmold on lettuce leaves and serve with lemon mayonnaise.

French Tomato Salad

Pour boiling water over medium-small, ripe tomatoes and drain immediately. Covering with cold water. Remove the skins and hollow out carefully. Fill the cavity with a mixture of chipped celery, finely diced cucumber, and tomato seasoned with Soy Mayonnaise and chopped parsley. Serve on a lettuce leaf.

Watercress Special Salad

Use equal parts of green onions, celery, green peppers, parsley, cucumbers and watercress — all diced, chopped, or minced as needed.

Mix and place a serving on lettuce leaves. If the cucumbers are nice, with a thin fresh skin, do not peel but wash well and cut in thin, round slices; or lengthwise and arrange with some radishes around and over the other vegetables. Serve with or without dressing.

Vegetable Salad

1 cup finely diced or grated carrots	1 green pepper cut in thin rings or fine slices
1 cup finely diced celery	1 cup finely cut parsley
1 cup cabbage chopped fine	

Mix the carrots, celery, and cabbage together and put as large a serving as you wish on lettuce leaves, arranging the rings or slices of green pepper around the mixed vegetables. Garnish with whole sprigs of parsley. Chopped nuts sprinkled over this makes a very nourishing salad.

Soy Mayonnaise is very nice with this salad. A few olives arranged around or over it are an attraction.

Tossed Garden Salad

Use any chopped, raw vegetables such as lettuce torn into small pieces, radishes sliced, cucumber and or celery chopped, adding a bit of grated onion if you like. You might add a bit of chipped cauliflower, or even tender green peas or beans.

Try various kinds of lettuce and other green, leafy vegetables, or bring in some tender green leaves from your yard, such as cress or dandelion.

Serve with a simple dressing made of oil and lemon juice, seasoned with salt and honey or other natural sweetener and perhaps a dash of cayenne pepper.

Molded Vegetable Salad

7½ tablespoons lemon agar-agar	½ teaspoon salt
1⅔ cups boiling water	1 cup chopped cabbage
2 tablespoons lemon juice	½ cup chopped celery
2 tablespoons raw sugar (optional)	½ cup shredded carrots
	3 tablespoons chopped green peppers

Bring water to a boil and remove from stove, quickly adding agar-agar, lemon juice, sugar, and salt, and stir until dissolved.

Immediately stir in vegetables and pour into mold. Do not stir after mixture begins to set.

Cucumbers and green onions can be added to the mixture if desired; also chopped olives.

Mock Chicken Salad

2 cups vegetable loaf (see recipes)	3 tablespoons chopped ripe olives
1 cup chopped celery	1/2 cup Soy Mayonnaise
1/2 cup chopped toasted almonds	1 1/2 tablespoons lemon juice
	1/2 teaspoon soy sauce

Mix just before serving on salad greens. Top with sprinkle of paprika.

Sauté vegetable loaf. Combine Soy Mayonnaise, lemon juice, and soy sauce

Herby Vegetable Salad

4 medium tomatoes	1 tablespoon raw sugar
1 medium onion	1 teaspoon salt
2 cucumbers	1/8 teaspoon oregano
1 green pepper	1/2 teaspoon sweet basil
2/3 cup oil	1/2 teaspoon sweet marjoram
1/4 cup lemon juice	

Combine oil and other dressing ingredients; slice or cut and mix in vegetables. Chill for two hours, tossing now and then. You may add any other savory herbs or seasonings

Golden Cole Slaw

1 cup shredded rutabaga	1 cup shredded carrots
1 cup shredded cabbage	Watercress
Chopped onion to taste	

Mix vegetables very lightly together and serve with Soy Mayonnaise or other light dressing.

Fruit Salad

In making fruit salads be careful of your combinations. Citrus fruits do not combine well with other fruits such as dates or figs. Avocados may be used with citrus fruits. Combine avocados as you wish using figs and dates as a garnish. When using avocados drop some lemon juice over them. Any kind of nuts may be used with a fruit salad. A sprinkling of finely ground nuts makes the salad more nourishing.

Good Combinations For Fruit Salads

Thompson seedless grapes, fresh peaches, diced cantaloupe.

Ripe bananas, fresh coconut (shredded or ground), cherries, pineapple.

Bananas, apples, pineapple.

Apples, raisins, walnuts.

Ripe strawberries, ripe bananas.

Red raspberries, bananas.

Black raspberries, bananas.

Ripe pears, strawberries, bananas.

Fresh coconut is a good combination with any fresh fruit.

All berries and fruits must be vine-ripened and tree-ripened to be really valuable for food. Be careful that bananas are fully ripened; they must not show any green on the ends and must be sprinkled with black spots before they are really ripe and valuable for food.

Fruit salads look nice served on fresh, crisp lettuce leaves but it would be better not to eat the lettuce with the fruits.

Soy Mayonnaise diluted to the consistency of cream is delicious with fruit salads.

Apple-Raisin Salad

1/2 cup whole wheat flakes	1/2 cup diced or chopped
1/2 cup chopped raisins	raw apples

It is best to soak the raisins overnight before using. More or less of any ingredient may be used to suit the convenience and taste. Mix ingredients together and serve. This makes a salad that anyone can live on.

Ambrosia

Grapefruit sections	Orange sections
Crushed pineapple	Grapes
Bananas	Strawberries
Cherries	

Mix together, chill, and serve in dessert cups.

Stuffed Date Salad

Remove pits from washed dates. Fill each date with half a walnut meat and press together. Put into a salad bowl and wet with lemon juice. Serve on a lettuce leaf.

Vegetables

Be sure to read the good advice on cooking vegetables in the first chapter. Their value to your good health depends first of all on having good produce, grown naturally; then on how fresh it is when you prepare it; then on how you cook it.

Here are some brief directions for the simplest preparation of some basic vegetables, probably more healthful served plain than in more complex dishes.

Baked Potatoes

Select smooth, medium-sized potatoes, wash, and prick with a fork all over to let moisture escape. Bake in a hot oven for 40 to 60 minutes. Serve as soon as done, with Soy Butter (see recipe).

Mashed Potatoes

Boil or steam potatoes with skins on until done. Remove skins, mash, season with salt and rich Soy Milk (see recipe), put in moderate-to-hot oven for half an hour and serve at once.

Boiled Cabbage

Select a head of cabbage that has as many of the outside green leaves on as are fit to use. Slice in eighths, put in a cooking pan and cover with sliced onion. Pour boiling water over it and cook for about 20 minutes or until tender. Salt when about half done.

Carrots and Peas

Equal parts of carrots and peas can be cooked together until tender and seasoned with rich Soy Milk or Soy Butter. Salt to taste.

String Beans

Wash, string, and break beans about one-half inch long or slice lengthwise. Cover bottom of pan with a little oil and put beans in pan. Salt, cover pan with a tight lid and cook until the beans are a bright green, stirring often so they will not stick. Then add a small amount of boiling water and cook until tender, watching carefully to avoid burning. Just before serving, stir in Soy Butter to taste.

Mixed Greens

Use as many kinds of greens as you wish, all as near the same tenderness as possible. Wash and chop. Rub kettle with a little garlic, add enough oil to just cover bottom of kettle, put the greens in, cover tightly, and cook about 10 minutes. Salt and serve at once.

Okra

Select even-sized, tender pods of okra. Cook until tender in just enough water to keep from burning. Salt and season with Soy Butter just before serving.

Spinach

Wash until thoroughly clean, put in a tightly covered kettle and cook until tender — from 5 to 10 minutes. Salt when partly done.

Jerusalem Artichokes

Select required number and peel. May be served raw or with Soy Mayonnaise.

Creamed Jerusalem Artichokes

Wash and peel the desired number of artichokes and cut them into half-inch cubes. Cook these in boiling, salted water until tender enough to be pierced with a fork. Drain and serve with hot cream sauce (see recipes).

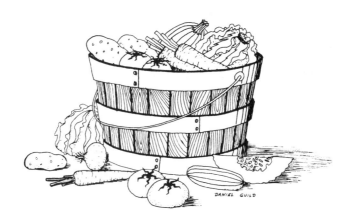

Cabbage Rolls With Dressing

Use one tender cabbage leaf per serving. Pour boiling water over them, then boil for three minutes and drain.

To half a cup of bread crumbs add a medium-sized onion chopped fine, one medium-sized grated carrot, and one-half cup chopped nuts. Add a little tomato juice and whatever seasoning is desired.

On each cabbage leaf place a large tablespoonful of the dressing and roll it up. Place the cabbage rolls in a baking dish with a little water or tomato juice in the bottom. Bake for 30 minutes in moderate oven. Serve with chopped parsley.

Scalloped Cabbage

4 cups cooked cabbage	1 teaspoon salt
1 cup bread crumbs	1/2 cup Soy Milk (see recipe)
2 tablespoons flour	1/2 cup water
1/2 cup liquid from cabbage	

Put one-fourth of the crumbs on the bottom of a baking dish. Shred the cabbage and put half of it over the crumbs. Add another fourth of the crumbs and the remaining cabbage. Over all this pour a white sauce (flour, salt, Soy Milk, water, and liquid from the cabbage). Sprinkle the rest of the crumbs over the top. Bake in a slow oven until thoroughly heated

Baked Carrots

10 medium-sized carrots	1 teaspoon salt
1/2 minced onion	3 tablespoons oil
1/2 cup minced parsley	1/3 cup boiling water
1 tablespoon brown sugar	

Wash and scrape carrots lightly; cut in half — lengthwise and crosswise. Place in a baking dish. Mix the remaining ingredients. Sprinkle mixture over the carrots, then pour boiling water over all. Cover and bake in a moderate-to-hot oven about an hour and a half.

Quick and Easy Corn Chowder

1 large potato
1 onion
1 No. 2 can creamed corn

1 or 2 cups Soy Milk
  (see recipe)
Salt or other seasoning to taste

Scrape potatoes. Dice potatoes and onion. Cook for about 10 minutes in a little water. Add Soy Milk and seasonings. Heat and serve.

Stuffed Cucumbers

4 large cucumbers
2 cups boiled natural rice
1 tablespoon chopped onion
1 teaspoon salt

$1/4$ teaspoon Savory Seasoning
  (see recipe)
$1/2$ teaspoon finely chopped
  parsley

Cut peeled cucumbers in halves and remove pulp (a teaspoon will work fine). Place in slightly salted water. Rinse and put into boiling water for three minutes. Place in cold water. Drain.

Fill with the rice, seasoning, salt, and parsley.

Sauté the onions, then sprinkle with bread crumbs. Put on top of the filled cucumbers.

Cover and bake in hot oven until tender. Then remove cover to brown.

German Green Beans

2 cups fresh green beans
6 small white rose potatoes
3 cups Soy Milk

Savory Seasoning to taste
  (see recipe)

Wash and cut beans and place in a small amount of boiling water. Allow to cook while you wash and cut potatoes into eighths or dice in one-inch pieces. Add to beans and continue boiling in as little water as possible until potatoes are cooked.

Add milk and heat to serve.

Baked Eggplant Casserole

3 cups diced raw eggplant
    unpeeled
½ cup chopped onions
½ cup green peppers

2½ cups tomatoes
3 tablespoons oil
Salt
Garlic

Put onions and peppers in hot oil and brown slightly, add eggplant and garlic and cook a few minutes. Add tomatoes and bake about 30 minutes in a moderate-to-hot oven. If you peel the eggplant, do it very thinly.

Eggplant Croquettes

2 cups cooked mashed
    eggplant
⅓ cup diluted Soy Milk

¼ cup unbleached flour
¼ tablespoon celery salt
3 cups cracker crumbs

Combine ingredients, form into croquettes, and bake. Baste frequently with a mixture of water and oil.

Eggplant-Zucchini Casserole

2 pounds eggplant
2 pounds zucchini
1 pound green pepper

2 cups tomato juice
2 cloves garlic
Salt

Wash but do not peel vegetables, then dice them. Brown in heavy, heated pan, turning to prevent burning.

Add the other ingredients, cover, and cook at least 45 minutes or until eggplant is done. Add tomato juice as needed.

May be served hot or cold or reheated if desired. Green beans, cauliflower, and onions are all good additions.

Kohlrabi

Kohlrabi is the "cabbage-turnip" with its nutrients stored in the bulb-like growth just above the ground. Should be used when it is not more than two or three inches in diameter. If larger, it is likely to be tough and fibrous.

Wash, pare thinly, and cut in thin slices. Place in slightly salted boiling water and boil partially covered until tender.

Drain, mash or dice, and season with a little rich Soy Cream or oil and salt, if desired.

The tops can be chopped, cooked separately as greens, then added to the mashed or diced root.

Savory Okra

1 quart okra	½ small onion
2 cups diced celery	4 tablespoons oil
1 sweet green pepper	2 large tomatoes, or 2 cups
Salt to taste	canned tomatoes

Cut okra crosswise in ¼-inch pieces and mix with celery. Steam until tender. Sauté the pepper and onion in the oil. Add the finely diced tomatoes and salt. Combine with the okra and celery. Stew for a few minutes to blend the flavors and serve hot.

Baked Onions With Mushrooms and Peas

6 large onions	2 tablespoons oil
¾ cup sliced mushrooms	1¼ cups Soy Milk
½ cup peas	(see recipe)
½ tablespoon salt	1½ tablespoons flour

Peel the onions and cut a thick slice from top of each. Scoop out center. Cook covered in small quantity of water until tender.

Fill the cooked onion cups with the following mixture.

Make a sauce with oil and flour, add milk and stir until smooth. Salt. Add sautéed mushrooms and peas. Sprinkle with chopped parsley and serve hot.

Corn-Onion Casserole

2 cups thinly sliced onions	2 tablespoons chopped
1½ cups whole kernel corn	pimiento
1 tablespoon oil	Salt to taste

Green Peas in a Cup

Wash medium-sized turnips and hollow them out, about one-fourth inch thick. Cook in boiling, salted water until tender but still firm. Fill with hot, cooked peas, and cover with a milk sauce (see recipes).

Bake the sliced onions in covered, oiled baking dish until just tender. Stir in corn and pimiento. Return to oven long enough to steam through. Season and serve.

Creamed Peas On Toast

³/₄ cup green pea pulp	¹/₄ cup thin Soy Cream
Salt to taste	(see recipe)

Add hot Soy Cream to cooked washed peas and salt to taste. Reheat. Dip a piece of zwieback in hot Soy Milk to soften, cover with creamed peas (should be thick enough to stay on toast).

Green Peas With Mushrooms

¹/₂ cup green peas	1 teaspoon seasoned salt
2 teaspoons chopped onion	¹/₂ teaspoon Savory Seasoning
2 4-ounce cans sliced	(see recipe)
mushrooms with liquid	2 tablespoons oil

Combine all ingredients in saucepan, cover, and bring to a boil. Reduce to low heat and cook four to six minutes only. Drain and serve.

Stuffed Green Peppers

2 cups soybean pulp	1 cup celery
³/₄ teaspoon salt	¹/₂ cup tomatoes
1 teaspoon chopped onion	

Remove the inside material from eight green peppers and boil them for three minutes. Sprinkle inside with salt. Fill with mixture of bean pulp, celery, tomatoes, and onion and cover with oiled crumbs. Place in oiled pan and bake in moderate oven 20 to 30 minutes, or until peppers are soft.

Cooking Potatoes

We hear so much about mashed potatoes not being good to eat. It is true that the ordinary mashed potatoes as they are eaten everywhere are very poor food. When potatoes are peeled, boiled, and mashed with a large piece of butter or other fat they become unwholesome. When potatoes are peeled there is almost nothing left but starch. The alkaline part of the potato is cut away, leaving the acid-forming sarch.

I must mention again that the eyes and the peeling of the Irish potato contain its life-giving properties. When the skin of the potato is not eaten the best part of it is lost. Also, when the skin is baked too brown the life-giving properties are destroyed.

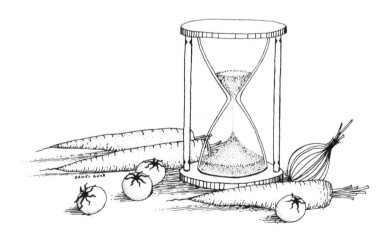

Baking is the ideal way to cook potatoes but it must be properly done. When properly baked the skin should be a little crisp but not too brown or black. Before putting potatoes in the oven to bake (after they have been thoroughly scrubbed) prick them all over with a fork. This causes some of the moisture to evaporate and helps to make them dry and mealy.

Another excellent way to prepare potatoes is to steam cook or pressure cook them. All vegetables may be well-prepared in the steam pressure cooker under a low temperature with the original food flavors preserved in an economical way. They can be further improved by placing them in an oven and allowing them to dry out for a few minutes. Many who have found it impossible to eat potatoes prepared in other ways can eat them prepared this way.

Mashed Potatoes

Select the dry, mealy variety of potato, such as Idaho. Wash them thoroughly and boil or steam until they are thoroughly done. Steaming is best. When done, peel the outer thin skin off, being careful not to remove the eyes. Mash, add rich Soy Milk and salt to taste. Bake for 20 minutes in a hot oven.

Scalloped Potatoes

Thinly peel raw potatoes and slice thin. Put a layer of the slices into an oiled baking pan and sprinkle with salt and flour. Make other layers until the pan is about three-fourths full. Pour enough Soy Milk over the potatoes to cover. Bake until thoroughly done. The dish may be garnished with chopped nuts.

Stuffed Baked Potatoes

Bake six large Idaho potatoes (with unbroken skin). After removing from the oven, rub with oil and cut in half, lengthwise. Scrape out the pulp carefully and mash. Take 1 teaspoon Savory Seasoning (see recipe) dissolved in hot Soy Milk that has been diluted (half hot water and half milk). Moisten pulp with hot, diluted Soy Milk, seasoned with Savory Seasoning and salt. Beat until light, then fill each potato shell. Sprinkle with finely chopped nuts and bake until light brown.

Stuffed Sweet Potatoes

4 medium-sized sweet potatoes	¹/₄ teaspoon salt
²/₃ cup Soy Milk (see recipe)	¹/₃ cup chopped peanuts
¹/₄ cup peanut butter	Seasonings to taste

Cut hot baked sweet potatoes in half and carefully remove from shells. Leave shells whole. Mash sweet potato thoroughly, mix with milk, peanut butter, and seasonings. Beat until fluffy, refill shells.

Sprinkle chopped nuts on top and brown on a baking sheet in a hot oven.

New England Boiled Dinner

4 medium-sized potatoes	¹/₂ small cabbage
4 small carrots	1¹/₂ tablespoon oil
4 turnips	Salt to taste
6 small onions	

Cut the peeled carrots and turnips into quarters. Add whole onions and put into a saucepan with moderate amount of water. Add the salt, cover, and bring to a boil. Separate the leaves of the cabbage and steam separately for five minutes. Drain and add to the vegetables.

When the carrots are about half cooked, add the potatoes cut into halves, and the oil. Salt to taste and let cook slowly until thoroughly done.

Serve with the cabbage in the center of the platter and other vegetables arranged attractively around it.

Baked Stuffed Squash

6 medium-sized round summer squash	1 cup of grated Soy Cheese (see recipe)
2 cups bread crumbs	4 tablespoons oil

Wash squash and boil whole in salted water until tender. Cut in half and scoop out pulp. Mix pulp with crumbs and fill shells. Sprinkle with Soy Cheese and bake in moderate oven until brown.

Flavorful Swiss Chard

2 bunches Swiss chard	1 teaspoon Soy Butter
1½ medium-sized onions	8 tomatoes
Salt	

Wash the chard, cut into a pan, cover and put directly into the oven. It will cook without added water.

Simmer the other ingredients slightly in a skillet and mix with the chard.

Baked Breaded Tomato

Fill a flat, shallow baking dish about three-fourths full of stewed or sliced raw tomatoes. Add 2 tablespoons chopped onion, 1 tablespoon honey. Add salt if using raw tomatoes.

Spread whole wheat bread with Soy Butter (see recipe) and place on tomatoes buttered side up.

Bake covered until tomatoes are done then remove cover to brown the bread.

Hashed Brown Potatoes

3 cups finely cooked potatoes	1 or 2 tablespoons minced onion
3 tablespoons soy flour	
3 tablespoons oil	½ cup rich Soy Milk
	1 teaspoon salt

Heat oil in skillet; add potatoes. Combine flour, onion,

milk, and salt in a small bowl and pour over potatoes. Place skillet over medium heat and cook 10 minutes without turning. Turn once and cook on other side until brown.

Dixieland Potpourri

VEGETABLES

2 cups green peas	3 small yellow squash
2 cups green beans	3 small zucchini
1 head cauliflower	1 cup celery
1 cup carrots	1 cup diced green pepper
1 cup okra	1 large Bermuda onion
1 cup corn kernels	3 medium tomatoes

SEASONINGS

1 cup hot water (or vegetable broth on hand, such as potato water)	2 tablespoons olive oil
	3 cloves garlic, diced
	1 bay leaf, small pieces
2 teaspoons Savory Seasoning (see recipe)	1 teaspoon salt
	3 tablespoons parsley

Preheat oven to 350 degrees.

Dissolve Savory Seasoning in hot liquid in saucepan. Add all seasonings. Bring to boil and simmer while preparing vegetables, adding small amount of hot water if too much evaporates. Onions and garlic can be simmered in this with seasonings.

Separate cauliflower into flowerets, and slice onion thinly. All other larger vegetables should be sliced in half-inch slices. (Diagonal slices make the dish more attractive, or using a variety of shapes adds interest.)

Put vegetables in ungreased baking dish, either casserole or earthenware pot, and mix together. Pour hot sauce mixture over vegetables, cover tightly and bake for one hour or until tender.

Other vegetables may be substituted and any that are not liked may be eliminated. The same is true with the seasonings.

Baked Lima Beans In Tomato Sauce

1 cup dry lima beans
2 small onions
1 tablespoon tomato paste

Salt to taste
1/4 cup brown sugar
2 tablespoons oil

Cover lima beans with plenty of water and soak overnight. Do not throw water away — use it to cover beans in baking dish. Add oil and salt to beans and cook until tender (not mushy). Simmer onions until tender. Then put beans in baking dish and add sugar, tomato paste, and simmered onions. Bake in hot oven for about one hour.

Eggplant Surprise

1 large eggplant
1/4 cup chopped onion
1/2 cup chopped green pepper
3 tablespoons oil

1 1/2 cups tomato juice
1 tablespoon cornstarch
1 teaspoon salt

Cut top off eggplant; reserve to use as lid. Scoop out pulp to within half inch of skin; reserve eggplant shell to use as a serving dish. Dice pulp. Parboil for five minutes. Drain. Cook onion and pepper in oil until lightly browned. Combine with eggplant pulp, soup and seasonings. Bake, uncovered, in moderate oven for 45 minutes.

Before serving, fill eggplant shell with boiling water; let stand five minutes. Drain. Fill with baked eggplant mixture. Cover with eggplant lid.

Sauces
Seasonings, Spreads

Many otherwise wholesome foods are ruined by smothering them with starchy sauces seasoned with harmful condiments and heavy with hard-to-digest fats.

The best foods of all are the simplest — raw or cooked as little as possible, with only such oil and seasonings really required in order to be palatable.

But because some sauces and seasonings are desired in many homes and because they can be made not only palatable but wholesome, we have included these recipes. Some of them are specified in other recipes in this book.

Soy Gravy

Into one quart boiling Soy Milk, add oatmeal flour or quick oats to make the desired consistency. Oatmeal flour works faster.

Let simmer until thickened, stirring with a pancake turner so it will not burn on the bottom. Add a little soy sauce or Vegetable Extract to lend a meaty flavor.

This gravy may be made with water instead of milk and enriched with a little Soy Butter and a little fine-cut onion.

Savory Oatmeal Gravy

1 quart boiling water	Vegetable Extract to taste
4 ounces oatmeal flour or quick oats	Salt
1 tablespoon oil	Bay leaf, onion, or other desired flavoring.

Into boiling water stir gradually the oatmeal flour or oats. Boil until thickened. Add the oil and seasoning.

This makes a very wholesome and well-flavored gravy.

Plain Brown Gravy

1/2 tablespoon oil	1 3/4 cups warm water
1/3 cup flour	1/4 teaspoon salt

Heat the oil, stir in flour, remove from heat. Gradually add the water, stirring until smooth. Cook for 5 to 10 minutes.

Healthful Ketchup

1 quart tomatoes	4 tablespoons natural sugar
1 medium onion	1 1/2 teaspoons salt
1 large stalk celery	1 teaspoon Savory Seasoning (see recipe)
1/2 green pepper or pimiento	1 bay leaf
1 clove garlic or garlic salt	1 teaspoon basil
3 sprigs parsley	2 tablespoons lemon juice
3 ounces tomato paste	

Chop onion, celery, pepper, parsley, garlic and tomatoes and cook until tender. Put through a food grinder. Add other ingredients — the lemon juice last. Bring to boil. It is then ready for use or canning.

Malt Honey

To 1 pound of wheat or corn meal, add 8 quarts of water. Boil until it thickens (so that the starch is cooked). Cool to between 140°F and 170°F, then add 2 ounces of barley malt, either in powder or syrup form. Stir. Let stand until the starch is changed into dextrose or malt honey. When the water is clear, pour or siphon it off, being careful not to get any mash from the bottom; otherwise the Malt Honey will not be clear. Now boil it down to the consistency of syrup.

Milk Sweetening

1 cup Malt Honey (see above)   1 cup oil

Slowly pour oil into the Malt Honey, beating constantly. In this way the fat is emulsified and easily digested.

Soy Mayonnaise

1 heaping tablespoon
   fineground soy flour
½ pint cold water
½ pint soy oil

1 tablespoon lemon juice
   (more or less to taste)
Pinch of salt

The addition of paprika or cayenne is healthful.
Color with a pure vegetable butter coloring.
Mix the soy flour into the cold water, boil for five minutes. Cook in a smooth, flat-bottomed dish; stirring with a pancake turner to keep free from the bottom of the dish as it burns very quickly.

Strain through a fine sieve into a medium-sized mixing bowl. While beating rapidly and continuously (or using a blender) pour in the soy oil in a very fine stream. If the oil is poured in fast, the mayonnaise will separate after standing a while. (If this should happen, pour the oil off and beat again.) It will be very simple after you have made it a few times.

Add salt, coloring, paprika and cayenne, and beat just enough to mix well. It needs only a small pinch of cayenne to make it taste snappy.

Use more or less soy oil to make it any consistency you wish. Peanut oil may be used in place of soy oil.

A clove of garlic cut and rubbed on the bowl in which the mayonnaise is made greatly adds to the flavor.

This mayonnaise can be used anywhere that dairy cream is used. It makes a very fine dressing for cole slaw or any kind of greens.

Dixie Mayonnaise

Dilute ½ cup raw peanut butter with 1 cup of water. Beat in 1 cup of oil and add about 1 tablespoon lemon juice. Salt to taste.

This can also be boiled for two or three minutes, then beaten thoroughly.

Quick Soy Mayonnaise

½ cup water	¼ teaspoon paprika
¼ cup soy milk powder	½ cup oil (scant)
¼ teaspoon salt	Juice of 1 lemon

Put water in blender and blend in soy milk powder and seasonings. Add the oil slowly at high speed. Remove from blender and add the lemon juice, more or less according to taste.

White Sauces

For **Very Thin Sauce**, use 1 cup Soy Milk, ½ tablespoon oil, ½ tablespoon unbleached flour. This sauce is used in making cream soups.

For **Thin Sauce**, use 1 cup Soy Milk, 1 tablespoon oil, 1 tablespoon unbleached flour. This sauce is also used for cream soups.

For **Medium Sauce**, use 1 cup Soy Milk, 2 tablespoons oil, 2 tablespoons unbleached flour. This sauce may be used for creaming vegetables and for gravies.

For **Thick Sauce**, use 1 cup Soy Milk, 2 to 3 tablespoons oil, 2½ tablespoons unbleached flour. This sauce may be used for heavy gravies and puddings.

Paste Sauce

1 cup Soy Milk	4 tablespoons unbleached
4 tablespoons oil	flour

This is used in soufflés. For method of making see below.

Heavy Paste Sauce

1 cup Soy Milk	6 tablespoons unbleached
4 to 6 tablespoons oil	flour

This sauce is used in croquettes.

Blend oil and flour in double boiler. Add the liquid. Fruit juice may be substituted for the Soy Milk. Stir until smooth and done. Salt to taste. With tomato juice, seasoned with onion and pimiento, this makes a good Spanish sauce.

Herb Sauce

1 tablespoon Savory Seasoning (see recipe)	1/2 teaspoon ground sage
1 tablespoon grated onion	1 tablespoon chopped parsley
1 bay leaf	1 tablespoon vegetable butter
1 tablespoon unbleached flour	1 tablespoon lemon juice
2 cups strained tomato	1/4 cup vegetable broth (from cooking vegetables)
1 tablespoon celery salt	

Sauté onion, bay leaf, butter and parsley. Remove the bay leaf when flavored to taste. Add liquids and bring to a boil. Thicken with flour.

Mushroom Sauce

1 1/2 cups coarsely chopped mushrooms	1 teaspoon soy sauce
1/3 cup diced gluten	1 1/2 tablespoons pimiento
1/2 cup browned flour	1 1/2 cups hot Soy Milk
1 1/2 tablespoons oil	Salt to taste

Blend oil and flour, then stir in the hot milk slowly until smooth. Add the soy sauce, pimiento, and salt. Cook 5 to 10 minutes, then stir in mushrooms and gluten. (These should be browned first in a little oil.)

Parsley Sauce

Chop fresh parsley and add enough parsley to the recipe for White or Paste Sauce.

Creole Sauce

2 cups stewed tomato	1½ tablespoons oil
½ cup diced onion	A sprinkle of natural sugar
½ cup diced green pepper	Salt to taste
1 clove garlic	Chopped parsley

Put oil, pepper, onion, and crushed garlic into a saucepan, cover, and simmer for a few minutes, stirring often. Add the tomato and boil gently for 10 or 15 minutes. Add salt to taste; the sweetening, and chopped parsley.

Quick Spaghetti Sauce

Sauté chopped green peppers, onions, and mushrooms in a little oil. Add a little sauce.

Add to this mixture a sauce prepared as follows: mash a can of tomatoes in saucepan, season with salt, garlic, celery salt, and smoke flavoring if you like. Simmer a while then combine with mixture above and simmer together for about half an hour. Serve over cooked spaghetti of good quality.

Vanilla Sauce

To Soy Cream you may add malt sugar or honey and vanilla. This makes a delicious sauce to be used in place of starchy sauces or whipping cream.

Savory Seasoning

$^{1}/_{2}$ cup tomato juice
$^{1}/_{2}$ cup soy sauce
1 cup brewer's yeast

Seasonings desired such
as garlic, onion

Put juice and soy sauce in pan and add seasonings. Bring to boil and remove at once from fire. Add the brewer's yeast and stir until smooth. Add more yeast if necessary to make right consistency.

Vegetable Extract

1 pound compressed yeast
1 tablespoon salt

$^{1}/_{4}$ cup strong Cereal Coffee
(see recipe)

Boil about five minutes. Amounts may be altered in proportion to make the amount of extract you want.

Mild Vegetable Extract

1 pound compressed yeast
1 teaspoon Vegetable
Extract above

1 tablespoon salt
2 tablespoons water

Boil until it thickens. Amounts may be altered in proportion to make the amount of extract you want.

Desserts for Health

Our appetites seem to call for a touch of sweetness with a meal. Although good health can be maintained without desserts — more easily than with them — we offer some recipes that provide a delicious sweetness in the menu but avoid the heavy fats, starches, and spices that make ordinary desserts so hard on the system.

Apples

The apple is rightly called the King of Fruits. Those who have too much acid may benefit from sweet apples, which have little acid, and those who have not acid enough can benefit from sour apples. Old people and very small babies can eat a mellow apple, if it is scraped, and do well on it.

Apples are very high in food value, in life-giving properties. They should not be eaten between meals but one can make an entire meal of them. If you have good teeth eat the peeling, core, and seeds and chew them thoroughly. Apple is especially good for diabetes and is also excellent for the liver and kidneys as well as being beneficial in correcting hyper-acidity.

An exclusive apple diet for a while would prove of great benefit to the system. A glass of good apple juice an hour before each meal would prove of great benefit but it must be made from good, sound apples. Ordinary apple cider is not fit to be used.

Baked Apples

Wash the apples and remove the cores, leaving apples whole. Fill the place from which cores were removed with raisins or dates and bake in a flat baking dish with a little water in bottom. Nut meats may also be used with raisins for added flavor Serve with Nut Cream (see recipe).

Baked Honey Apples

4 apples	1 tablespoon lemon juice
1/3 cup honey	1 cup boiling water

Wash and core the apples, and place in a baking pan. Fill holes with thick honey. Add lemon juice to water and pour into pan. Bake for 15 minutes in a moderate oven, basting several times.

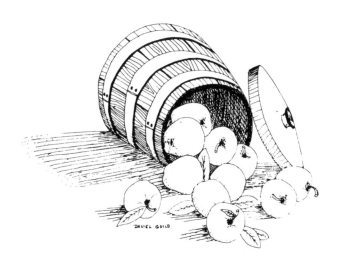

Scalloped Apples

4 cups thinly sliced apples
3 tablespoons Nut Butter
  (see recipe)
1/2 cup honey

3 cups soft whole wheat
  bread crumbs
1/3 cup water

Blend and bake in moderate oven for 20 minutes.

Easy Apple Sauce

4 quarts apple pieces

2 cups honey

Add just enough water to the apples to prevent them from sticking to the pan. Simmer until tender. Mash through a sieve. Add honey while sauce is warm and blend thoroughly.

Apple Crisp

6 cups thinly sliced apples
6 tablespoons honey
2 teaspoons oil
1/2 teaspoon salt
6 tablespoons Soy Cream
  or Soy Butter

2/3 cup natural sugar
2 tablespoons whole wheat
  flour
3 cups wheat flakes or
  flaked oats

Mix the apples, honey, oil, and salt. Pour into a baking dish and set aside.

To the Soy Cream or Soy Butter add sugar, flour, and flakes. Spread over apples. Cover and bake in moderate oven for 30 minutes. Remove cover and bake another 15 minutes or until apples are tender.

Saucy Apple Crisp

4 cups sliced apples
1 teaspoon cinnamon
1/2 teaspoon salt
1 cup brown sugar

1/4 cup water
3/4 cup sifted unbleached flour
1/3 cup oil

Place apple slices in a baking dish and sprinkle with cinnamon, salt, and water. Rub together the flour, oil, and brown sugar; then drop the mixture over the apple slices. Bake in a moderate oven for about 40 minutes.

Fresh Peach Crisp

8 large firm ripe peaches	³/₄ cup brown sugar,
¹/₄ cup raw sugar	firmly packed
¹/₄ teaspoon salt	¹/₂ cup oil
1 teaspoon lemon juice	¹/₂ cup chopped walnuts
³/₄ cup unsifted unbleached flour	

Peel, pit, and cut peaches into ³/₄-inch slices (should make about 5 or 6 cups). Mix the raw sugar and salt. Place a layer of peach slices in a baking pan and sprinkle with raw sugar and salt mixture; repeat layers with all the peaches and sugar. Sprinkle with lemon juice.

Combine flour, brown sugar, and oil. Mix in nuts. Sprinkle this mixture over the peaches. Bake in a moderate oven until top is browned (about 45 minutes).

Brown Betty

1 tablespoon lemon juice	¹/₄ teaspoon salt
1 cup whole wheat	1 quart chopped apples
zwieback crumbs	1 scant cup brown sugar
1¹/₂ cups seedless raisins	

Spread half the raisins over the bottom of a baking dish. Cover raisins with half the chopped apples. Sprinkle over the apples half the sugar and half the crumbs. Sprinkle over this the remainder of the raisins. Sprinkle on the rest of the sugar and crumbs.

Add salt and lemon juice to ¹/₂ cup of water and pour this over top of pudding, set in a pan of water, cover and bake an hour. Remove from the pan of water and bake without the cover long enough to brown the top slightly. Serve with Vanilla Sauce (see below).

Vanilla Sauce

To the required amount of Soy Cream you may add malt sugar or honey and vanilla. This makes a delicious sauce to be used in the place of starchy sauces and whipping cream.

Indian Summer Pudding

1/3 cup corn meal	1/2 cup honey or maple syrup
2 1/2 cups Soy Milk	1/2 teaspoon salt
2 1/2 cups water	

Mix the corn meal with part of the Soy Milk. Mix the remainder of the milk and water in a double boiler, bring just to the boiling point, and add the corn meal. Add the honey and salt and cook for 15 or 20 minutes in the double boiler.

Pour into an oiled baking dish and bake in a very slow oven for about two hours. Serve with Soy Cream.

Rice Pudding

1 cup Soy Cream	1 cup cooked natural rice
Pinch of Salt	1 cup drained pineapple

Mix together, chill, and serve. Other fruits may be used in place of pineapple.

Nut-Rice Pudding

2 1/2 cups cooked brown rice	1 teaspoon grated orange rind
1 1/2 cups water	1 teaspoon grated lemon rind
1 cup raisins or chopped dates	1 teaspoon vanilla

Put 1 cup water in liquefier and liquefy with 1 cup cashews. Pour over rice. Rinse out liquefier with the other 1/2 cup water and add to rice. Add other ingredients and mix well. Bake in moderate oven 45 minutes to 1 hour. Serve hot or cold, plain or with Soy Cream.

Orange and Apple Tapioca Pudding

4 medium-sized tart apples	1/4 teaspoon salt
3/4 cup raw sugar	1/2 cup water
3 tablespoons oil	1 cup fresh or canned orange
1 tablespoon lemon juice	or tangerine sections
1/2 teaspoon cinnamon	1/4 cup tapioca (quick)
2 cups apple juice or water	

Peel the apples thinly; cut in pieces. Mix the pieces with the oil, sugar, lemon juice, cinnamon, salt, and water in a skillet; cover.

Over medium heat, bring to a boil; reduce heat and cover. Simmer for 15 minutes or so. Baste the apples now and then with the sugar mixture.

Remove apples (drained) to a serving dish and combine with orange sections.

Add tapioca and apple juice (or water) to the sugar mixture in the skillet. Let stand about five minutes. Bring to boil over medium heat, stirring constantly. Pour this mixture over the fruit and cool. After 20 minutes cooling, stir lightly and cool another 15 minutes or so before serving.

Soy Cream Tapioca

1/3 cup malt sugar or	1/2 cup tapioca
other natural sweetener	2 1/2 cups Soy Milk
1/3 cup Soy Cream	

Soak the tapioca in Soy Milk 15 minutes. Add the sugar, salt, and bring to a boil, stirring constantly. Place in a double boiler and cook until tapioca is transparent. Add vanilla, chill, and serve with Soy Cream.

Soy Ice Cream

2 quarts rich Soy Milk	1/2 pint Soy Butter
2 pounds malt sugar or	or Soy Mayonnaise
other natural sweetener	1 tablespoon agar-agar

Soak the agar-agar in cold water until it swells, drain and put in Soy Milk, add the sweetener and butter or mayonnaise. Fresh fruit or fruit juice may be added for flavoring, if desired. Refrigerate.

Vegetarian Gelatin

Soak 1 tablespoon of agar-agar in 1 pint warm water for 30 minutes. Drain and simmer 20 minutes in another pint of warm water and boil until dissolved. To this amount (which will be reduced by boiling) add, after straining, a pint of any desired fresh fruit or fruit juice. Bananas, peaches, or any other fresh fruit may be sliced in the bottom of each mold to give variety.

Before serving, decorate with crushed nut meats. For dressing, use Vanilla Sauce or Soy Cream.

Oatmeal Jell

1 quart water	Salt to taste
1 cup oatmeal	

Drop oatmeal very slowly into boiling salted water. Boil half an hour. Put through a sieve, turn into molds, and make cold. Serve with a little Malt Honey, honey, or fruit juice.

If a stiffer jell is desired, add a little agar-agar or Irish moss.

Soy Jelly

4 cups Soy Milk (unsweetened)	4 tablespoons malt sugar or
2 round tablespoons	other sweetening
agar-agar (flaky)	

Soak the agar-agar in the Soy Milk 1 hour. Put in a saucepan, bring to a boil, and simmer slowly until the agar-agar is entirely dissolved. Add the sweetening and cool.

Orange Jelly

1 cup malt sugar	³/₄ cup orange juice
other natural sweetener	³/₄ cup water
1 teaspoon grated orange rind	3 tablespoons lemon juice
1 tablespoon vegetable gelatin	

Mix the orange juice, rind, lemon juice, pinch of salt, and sweetening. Add the water. When boiled gelatin is ready, add the other ingredients, mold, and serve with Soy Cream.

Strawberry Jelly

1 tablespoon agar-agar	1 cup boiling water for agar
2 tablespoons lemon juice	1³/₄ cups crushed strawberries
1 cup malt sugar or	Few grains salt
natural sweetener	

Prepare as for Orange Jelly. When cool, decorate with strawberry halves and serve with crushed nuts or Soy Cream.

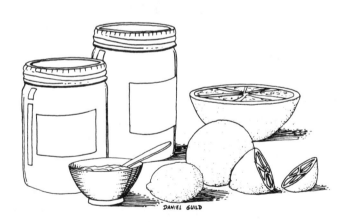

DANIEL GUILD

Fruit Pies

Fruit pies may be considered healthful when refined sugar is not used and when the crust is made of whole wheat flour and well-baked. Such a crust has a rich, nutty flavor and requires a little less shortening than when made of white flour. (Rich, starchy pie fillings and custards are among the most objectionable of all desserts.)

Unleavened Pie Crust

1 cup whole wheat flour
1 cup zwieback bread crumbs
2 tablespoons Soy Milk or oil

1 cup soy flour or
   soybean mash
Water or Soy Milk

Roll the zwieback bread crumbs with a rolling pin or run through a grinder. To the flour, crumbs, and soy flour or soybean mash, add the Soy Mayonnaise or oil.

Add the water or Soy Milk, making a dough stiff enough to be rolled and placed in pie tins. After it has been placed in a tin, place an empty tin inside, on top of the dough, and bake to a light brown before putting in the filling. After placing the filling in the crust, bake in a moderate oven for about 20 minutes.

This crust may be used for any kind of pie filling.

Raised Pie Crust

2 cups whole wheat flour
1 cup soy flour or soy mash
2 tablespoons malt sugar
   or honey

¼ yeast cake
2 tablespoons oil
Warm water

Dissolve the yeast in warm water and add the oil and sweetener. Now add the whole wheat flour and soy flour or soybean mash. Mix the same as bread dough and let rise for an hour or more in a warm place. When it has risen, knead down, and let rise 10 or 15 minutes. Then roll out thin and put in pie tins, allowing it to rise about 15 minutes.

Soybean Pumpkin Pie

1 cup mashed pumpkin
2 tablespoons fine zwieback
   crumbs
1/3 cup malt sugar, Malt
   Honey, or honey

2 cups hot Soy Milk
1/2 teaspoon, or less,
   vanilla or almond flavoring
A few grains of salt

Heat the milk. While the milk is heating, mix the zwieback crumbs, sweetener and salt. Stir them into the mashed pumpkin. Mix thoroughly and add the hot milk. Add seasoning. Pour into a crust and bake in a moderate oven until set.

Eggless Pumpkin Pie

2 cups pumpkin (or squash)
1/2 cup molasses
1/2 cup brown sugar
4 tablespoons whole
   wheat flour

2 cups rich Soy Milk
2 tablespoons honey
1 teaspoon cinnamon
Pinch of salt

Brown flour slightly in skillet. Combine ingredients and place in whole wheat pie crust to bake.

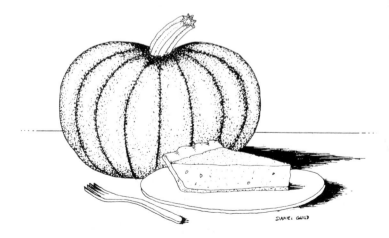

Banana-Prune Pie

1 pound cooked prunes	1/3 cup chopped nuts
2 bananas	1 tablespoon lemon juice
1 tablespoon cornstarch	1 teaspoon grated lemon rind

Remove pits from prunes; cut prunes in small pieces. Bring about 1 cup prune juice to a boil. Sweeten if desired and thicken with cornstarch. Add this — together with the chopped nuts, lemon juice, and lemon rind — to the prunes. Chill thoroughly. Just before serving, add sliced bananas and mix gently. Fill baked pie shell and top with Soy Cream.

Fig Marmalade Pie

1 cup figs	1 cup oil
1 cup pitted dates	3 tablespoons honey
1 cup raisins	3 cups Soy Milk

Mix and run through a food grinder. The holes in the plate of the grinder should be quite fine. This makes the fruit much easier to digest.

Reduce the thickness of the fruit mix with Soy Milk to the desired consistency. Turn this filling into a raised pie crust, directions for which are given in the foregoing recipes, and bake for 15 to 20 minutes in a moderate oven. No top crust is needed for this pie.

About 2 teaspoons of agar-agar may be added to the cold milk, soaked for a short time, and then boiled before adding to the fruit. This will help to thicken the filling.

Vanilla may be added for seasoning. This makes a very healthful pie, one that would be excellent in a school lunch for children. It is something they will like and which will nourish as well as satisfy them.

This pie filling may be prepared without the raisins. It may also be made with pitted dates alone, making a very sweet pie.

Old-fashioned turnovers may be made with this same filling.

Fruit and Nut Cookies

3 cups whole wheat flour
2 tablespoons sesame oil
½ cup honey
¼ cup chopped nuts

1 cup chopped mixed
  dried fruits
1 cup hot water

Add oil and honey to hot water. Stir in flour, nuts, and fruit. Drop by tablespoon onto cookie sheet. Bake in a moderate oven 45 minutes.

Diet Cookies

1 cup sesame meal or seeds
1 teaspoon salt
1½ small cans frozen,
  unsweetened orange juice

4 cups rolled oats
⅔ cups oil
1½ teaspoons vanilla

Place sesame meal or seeds in a heavy skillet until slightly brown.

Mix with oats and salt in large mixing bowl. Stir all

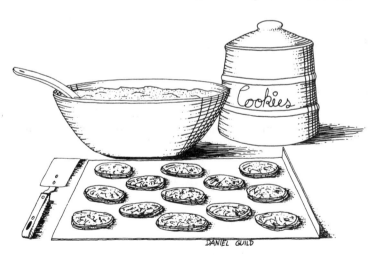

DANIEL GUILD

ingredients together and let stand 10 minutes. Drop by spoonful on baking sheet. Bake about 15 minutes in moderate oven.

Haystack Cookies

4 cups coconut	⅓ tsp salt
½ cup oatmeal	1⅓ cup water, cold
2⅓ cups walnuts, chopped	1½ cup peanut butter
5 cups dates, chopped	½ cup honey
1⅓ cup W. W. pastry flour	2 tsp vanilla

Mix all ingredients. Line sheet pans with baking paper (heavy wax paper). Use a level #20 ice cream scoop to place on pans, one scoop per cookie. Bake in 350 F. oven for 25 minutes or until light brown.

Sugarless Candy

1 cup coconut	½ cup toasted sesame seeds
1 cup soy milk powder	(or sunflower)
½ cup carob powder	¾ cup honey
1 cup chopped nuts	

Mix thoroughly, make into rolls, refrigerate, slice.

Carob Fudge

Cream ½ cup carob powder and ¼ cup margarine. Mix in ¼ cup honey, ½ cup soy milk powder, 1 cup nuts, and 1 teaspoon vanilla. Shape into roll and slice.

Delicious Dessert Sandwich

1 cup dates	1 cup raisins
1 cup figs	Juice of 2 oranges

Pit the dates and steam with other fruit until it is all soft. Mash thoroughly while adding orange juice. May be served hot or cold spread on thinly sliced whole wheat bread.

Coffees, Teas, Broths

Do not drink coffee and tea — they are harmful. Many herb drinks will satisfy just as well and with beneficial rather than harmful effects.

Take just one example — **peppermint tea**. Coffee weakens the heart muscles; peppermint tea is delicious and strengthens your heart muscles. Coffee hinders digestion, weakens the heart, is one cause of constipation, poisons the body. Peppermint tea cleanses and strengthens the entire body. Give it a fair trial and see how much better you feel when you leave off coffee and tea and drink peppermint tea.

In place of aspirin for a headache or any other harmful headache drug, take a cup of as-strong-as-you-like-it peppermint tea, lie down for a little while, and see what a good effect it will have. If need be, drink two or three cups, or enough so that it gets into the system so it can help you. It will not disappoint you. It strengthens the nerves instead of weakening them as aspirin and other drugs do.

If the tea is not at hand, take some of the leaves and chew them up fine until you can swallow them easily. This will start the food digesting and assist the entire system to do is work more normally.

Many Herb Teas

Numerous herbs can be used to make delicious beverages with good results for your health: red clover blossoms, sage, mint, sassafras, strawberry leaves, peppermint, spearmint, fennel, red raspberry leaves, hyssop, chickweed, catnip, wintergreen, sarsaparilla, wild cherry bark or small twigs, birch bark or small twigs, chicory, dandelion, yellow dock, camomile, hops, calamus root (sweet flag), meadow sweet, juniper berries, alfalfa, green celery leaves, horsemint, rue.

How To Make Herb Teas

To make teas from herbs, granulate them and use one heaping teaspoon (or if powdered, one-half teaspoon) to the cup of boiling water. Place the herbs in a pan and pour the boiling water over them. Then allow them to steep one-half hour. Cover. This steeping draws out of the herbs the mineral elements that are so beneficial to the system.

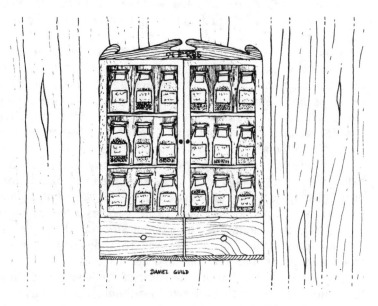

DANIEL GUILD

These teas are less expensiye than coffee and tea and they are healthful, not harmful.

You can read much more about them in the book **Back to Eden**, available from the publishers of this cookbook.

Soybean Coffee

Place the quantity of soybeans you desire in a dripping pan and heat in a hot oven, stirring frequently to prevent burning. The outside hull seems to brown less rapidly than the inner portion so you will find it necessary to take a few out occasionally and break them open with a hammer to see just how they are roasting.

To get a good flavored coffee, it is necessary to have an even roast. If part of the beans are not roasted quite enough and some a little too much, it spoils the flavor of the coffee.

After they are roasted, grind them through a course mill. Get some real coffee and compare the color so you will know how brown to make it. Half bran and half soybeans may also be used for a good coffee.

Rye Coffee

Cereal coffee can be made very easily at home.

Take the quantity of rye you desire and place in the oven in a dripping pan. Stir with a wooden paddle until the grain becomes as brown as coffee. Grind rather coarse in any little hand mill. It is now ready for use.

When roasting the whole grain it may help in checking on the browning process to take a little out with a spoon, lay it on a solid board, and break it up with a hammer for inspection.

Wheat Coffee

Wheat bran is used in this recipe. Mix equal parts water and Malt Honey (see recipe). Moisten the bran — a pound, or whatever quantity you desire — with the water and Malt Honey mixture. Let it get quite dry or altogether dry before roasting. You may use some other natural sweetener in place of Malt Honey.

It may be placed in the sun (or any place where it is airy) to dry so that it does not sour.

When dry, place in a hot oven in a dripping pan, stirring frequently until it is as brown as coffee. The flavor of this coffee is very pleasing.

Half bran and half rye may also be used. The rye, however, must be ground before mixing with the bran. This makes wheat coffee with a fine flavor.

Bran Water

To be used in any kind of soup stock, stew, or in any breads in place of ordinary water.

To 2 cups of bran, add 1 quart of water. Let it stand overnight. Strain through a fine sieve or cheesecloth.

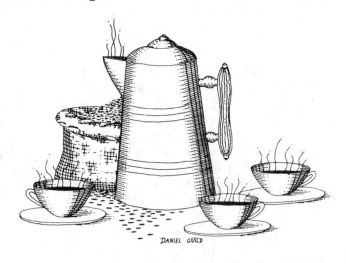

DANIEL GUILD

Bran Broth

Cook 1½ cups of the Bran Water (see above) for about five minutes. Add ½ cup of Soy Milk. More or less of the Bran Water and Soy Milk may be used; depending, of course, on the amount needed; but this is a good proportion to use. Season with Vegetable Extract (see recipe) and parsley.

Oatmeal Water

This is to be used in soup stocks, stew, or breads in place of water. It increases the vitamins and makes soups creamy.

To 1 quart of water, add 1 cup of oatmeal and soak overnight. Strain through a fine sieve or cheesecloth.

Oatmeal Broth

Prepare oatmeal water as given in the recipe above and cook five minutes. To each ¾ cup of oatmeal water, add ¼ cup Soy Milk. Season with Vegetable Extract (see recipe).

An excellent drink can also be made by using one part each of Bran Water and Oatmeal Water. Heat together, add Soy Milk, and season to taste. A little parsley, onion, or celery lends a pleasing flavor.

Herb Broth

Soak overnight 2 cups wheat bran in 1 quart of water, and 1 cup oatmeal in 1 quart of water. Stir up several times, then strain. Pour 1 pint of boiling water on 4 tablespoons of chickweek, let steep half an hour and strain. Mix the three ingredients together. Add 1 quart Soy Milk. Parsley, finely cut, may be added for flavoring; or season with celery or onions, as preferred. Let simmer for a few minutes and serve.

This broth contains all the ingredients the body requires.

Soybean Broth

Soak overnight 2 cups of wheat bran in 1 quart of unsweetened Soy Milk, and 1 cup of oatmeal in 1 quart of Soy Milk. In the morning, stir up several times, then strain.

Pour 1 pint of boiling, unsweetened Soy Milk on 4 heaping tablespoons of chickweed. Let stand for half an hour, then strain. Mix the three ingredients together, adding 1 quart unsweetened Soy Milk.

Add diced celery and onions for flavoring. Simmer together for 30 minutes, adding 3 tablespoons Soy Mayonnaise (see recipe). A few minutes before it is finished, add 1 cup of very finely cut parsley.

This broth contains all the ingredients the body requires.

Potassium Broth

Soak overnight 2 cups bran, 1 cup oatmeal, 4 quarts water. Beat with egg beater and strain through a fine sieve.

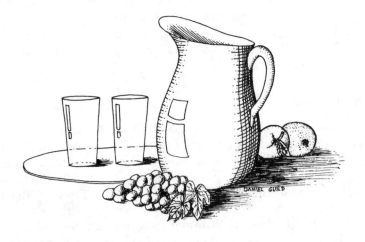

Wash thoroughly 4 medium-sized potatoes and slice thin; also 2 large carrots, 2 medium-sized onions (if onions are not liked, leave out), 2 large stalks celery cut fine with the green leaves, ½ bunch of chopped parsley, a few pieces of gluten (see recipe).

Cook together in the bran or oatmeal water.

Let simmer in covered kettle until vegetables are done, mash up vegetables, and strain again through fine sieve.

Tomato Nut Broth

3 cups stewed tomatoes	4 tablespoons chopped onion
2 tablespoons any kind of nut butter	1 large sprig parsley
4 cups vegetable broth (from cooking)	1 small bay leaf
	A sprinkle of thyme
	Salt

Put parsley, onion, bay leaf, and thyme into a small saucepan and let simmer for a few minutes. Add liquids and boil gently for 30 minutes. Add the nut butter, dissolved in warm water. Mix, salt, strain, and serve.

Index

Soy Milk, Cheese, Butter, and Cream

Soy Milk   35
Quick Soy Milk   36
How to Curd Soy Milk   37
Soy Buttermilk   37
Soy Butter   37
Soy Cream   37
Soy Cream Cheese   38
Soy Cottage Cheese   38
Soy Cheese   38
Quick Soy Cheese   39
Original Soy Cheese   39
Egg Yolk Substitute   40

Nut Milk, Cheese, Butter, and Cream

Nut Milk   41
Nut Cheese   41
Diet Nut Cheese   42
Malted Nut Cream   42
Superb Peanut Butter   43
Blanched Peanut Butter   43
Simple Nut Butter   43
Blanched Peanuts   43
Nut Meal   44
Nut Butter Cream   44

Main Dishes

Basic Wheat Protein (Gluten)   45
Peanut Gluten Roast   46
Protein Patties   46
Vegetable Sauerbraten
    with Noodles   47
Vegetable Potpie   47
Vegetable Salmon   47
Light and Delightful Peanut
    Butter Loaf   48
Soybean Loaf   48
Soy Cottage Cheese Loaf   49
German Cabbage Beroks   49
Italian Meat Balls   49
Nature's Own Meat Loaf   50
Peanut Roast   50
Tomato Loaf   51
Scotch Barley Roast   51
Lentil-Potato Roast   51
Savory Soy Loaf   52
Golden Nut Loaf   53

Vegetable Hash   53
Flavorful Nut and Potato Hash   53
Seasoned Lentil "Cutlets"   54
Lentil and Rice Loaf   54
Soy Patties   54
Nutty Lentil-Rice Loaf   55
Nut Loaf Orient   55
Italian Baked Rice   55
Seasoned Rice-Nut Patties   56
Southern Nut-Rice Loaf   56
Parsleyed Rice Meat Balls   56
Old-Fashioned Spanish Rice   57
Jerusalem Fillets   57
Vegetable Tamale   58
Beans, basic cooking methods   58
Sprouted Soybeans   58
Seasoned Soybeans   59
Southern Style Soybeans
Boston Baked Beans   59
Raw Spinach Sandwich   60
Toasted Tomato Sandwich   60

Using Sprouted Seeds

Sprouting methods   61
Sprouted Lentil Roast   62
Sprouted Soybeans with Rice   62
Soybean Sprout Salad   63
Vegetarian Chop Suey   63
Sprout Sandwich   64

Bread . . . a Health Food

Basic information on bread as food   65
Fermented and unfermented breads
Sponge bread   68
Yeast   68
Making bread rise   69
The oven   71
Old-fashioned clay oven   71
Using steam in the oven   73

Life-Giving Breads

Whole Wheat Bread   74
Rye Bread   75
Whole Wheat Raisin Bread
Steamed Whole Wheat Bread   76
Soybean Bread   77

Diet Soybean Bread   77
Soy Buns or Cinnamon Rolls   78
Sesame Cloverleaf Rolls   78
Old-Fashioned Beaten Biscuits   79
Corn Bread   80
Corn Pone   80
Special Corn Pone   81
Corn Dodgers   81
Zwieback   81
Health Muffins or Crackers   82
Unleaved Muffins   82
Cornmeal Muffins   83
Oatmeal or Soybean Muffins   83
Potato or Carrot Muffins   83
Olden Days Corn-Soy Muffins   84
Crisp Whole Wheat Crackers   84
Raised Oatmeal Crackers   85
Soy-Oat Crackers   85
Rye Crisps   85
Whole Wheat Sticks   85
Coconut-Wheat Sticks   86

Natural Breakfast Foods

Browned and Steamed Rice   87
Chinese Boiled Rice   87
Fluffy Soft Rice   88
Slow-Cooked Breakfast Rice   88
Soy Baked Rice   88
Breakfast Wheat   89
Cornmeal Mush   89
The Original Granola   90
Kloss' Granola   90
Granola Supreme   90
Old-Fashioned Granola   91
Original Dixie Kernel   91
Old-Fashioned Dixie Kernel   91
Kloss' Soy-Corn Pancakes   92
Kloss' Eggless French Toast   93

Soups . . . Total Nutrition

Bean Soup   94
Hot or Cold Borsch   95
Cream of Corn Soup   96
Eggplant Soup   96
Golden Soup   96
Cream of Lentil Soup   96
Rich Lentil Soup   97
Lentil-Herb Soup   97
Bean-Rich Minestrone   97
Cream of Lettuce and
   Poato Soup   98
Potato-Onion Soup   98
Cream of Spinach Soup   98
Old-Fashioned Stew   99
Tomato Soup   99

Rich Tomato Soup   99
Cream of Tomato Soup   100
Rich Cream of Tomato Soup   100
Pioneer Vegetable Soup   100
Robust Vegetable Soup   101
Year-Round Fruit Soup   102
Tropical Fruit Soup   102
Fresh Vegetable Minestrone   103
Grandmother Kloss'
   Split Pea Soup   103
Creamy Split Pea Soup   104
Rich Potato Soup   104

Salads and Dressings

Golden Salad Dressing   105
Green Pepper Salad Dressing   106
Lemon-Honey Dressing   106
Lemon-Honey French Dressing   106
Soy Salad Dressing   106
Sweet-and-Sour Dressing   106
Special Diet Dressing   107
Avocado-Stuffed Celery   107
Carrousel Bean Salad   107
Garden Salad   107
Lettuce Salad Rolls   108
Kloss' Potato Salad   108
High Protein Salad   109
Red, White, and Green Salad   109
Soybean Salad   109
Tomato Aspic Salad   110
French Tomato Salad   110
Watercress Special Salad   110
Vegetable Salad   110
Tossed Garden Salad   111
Molded Vegetable Salad   111
Mock Chicken Salad   112
Herby Vegetable Salad   112
Golden Cole Slaw   112
Good Combinations for
   fruit salads   113
Apple-Raisin Salad   113
Ambrosia   113
Stuffed Date Salad   114

Vegetables

Baked Potatoes   115
Mashed Potatoes   115
Boiled Cabbage   116
Carrots and Peas   116
String Beans   116
Mixed greens   116
Okra   116
Spinach   116
Jerusalem Artichokes   117
Creamed Jerusalem Artichokes   117

Cabbage Rolls with Dressing   118
Scalloped Cabbage   118
Baked Carrots   118
Quick and Easy Corn Chowder   119
Stuffed Cucumbers   119
German Green Beans   119
Baked Eggplant Casserole   120
Eggplant Croquettes   120
Eggplant-Zucchini Casserole   120
Kohlrabi   120
Savory Okra   121
Baked Onions with Mushrooms
    and Peas   121
Corn-Onion Casserole   121
Green Peas in a Cup   122
Creamed Peas on Toast   122
Green Peas with Mushrooms   122
Stuffed Green Peppers   122
How to cook potatoes   124
Scalloped Potatoes   124
Stuffed Baked Potatoes   124
Stuffed Sweet Potatoes   125
New England Boiled Dinner   125
Baked Stuffed Fquash   126
Flavorful Swiss Chard   126
Baked Stuffed Squash   126
Hashed Brown Potatoes   126
Dixieland Potpourri   127
Baked Lima Beans in
    Tomato Sauce   127
Eggplant Surprise   128

Sauces, Seasonings, and Spreads

Soy Gravy   129
Savory Oatmeal Gravy   130
Plain Brown Grayy   130
Healthful Ketchup   130
Malt Honey   130
Milk Sweetening   131
Soy Mayonnaise   131
Dixie Mayonnaise   132
Quick Soy Mayonnaise   132
White Sauces   132
Paste Sauce   133
Heavy Paste Sauce   133
Herb Sauce   133
Mushroom Sauce   133
Parsley Sauce   134
Creole Sauce   134
Quick Spaghetti Sauce   134
Vanilla Sauce   134
Savory Seasoning   135
Vegetable Extract   135
Mild Vegetable Extract   135

Desserts for Health

Apples, "King of Fruits"   136
Baked Apples   137
Baked Honey Apples   137
Scalloped Apples   138
Easy Apple Sauce   138
Apple Crisp   138
Saucy Apple Crisp   138
Fresh Peach Crisp   139
Brown Betty   139
Vanilla Sauce   140
Indian Summer Pudding   140
Rice Pudding   140
Nut-Rice Pudding   140
Orange and Apple Tapioca
    Pudding   140
Soy Cream Tapioca   141
Soy Ice Cream   141
Vegetarian Gelatin   142
Oatmeal Jelly   142
Soy Jelly   142
Orange Jelly   143
Strawberry Jelly   143
Fruit Pies   144
Unleavened Pie Crust   144
Raised Pie Crust   144
Soybean Pumpkin Pie   145
Eggless Pumpkin Pie   145
Banana-Prune Pie
Fig Marmalade Pie   146
Fruit and Nut Cookies   147
Diet Cookies   147
Haystack Cookies   148
Sugarless Candy   148
Carob Fudge   148
Delicious Dessert Sandwich   148

Coffees, Teas, and Broths

Peppermint Tea   149
Herb Teas, how to make   150
Soybean Coffee   151
Rye Coffee   151
Wheat Coffee   151
Bran Water   152
Bran Broth   153
Oatmeal Water   153
Oatmeal Broth   153
Herb Broth   153
Soybean Broth   154
Potassium Broth   154
Tomato Nut Broth   155